T0231253

Abuse of Older Men

Abuse of Older Men has been co-published simultaneously as *Journal of Elder Abuse & Neglect*, Volume 19, Numbers 1/2 2007.

Abuse of Older Men

Jordan I. Kosberg, PhD, ACSW
Editor

Abuse of Older Men has been co-published simultaneously as *Journal of Elder Abuse & Neglect*, Volume 19, Numbers 1/2 2007.

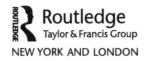

Routledge
Taylor & Francis Group
NEW YORK AND LONDON

First published by
The Haworth Press, Inc.
10 Alice Street
Binghamton, N Y 13904-1580

This edition published 2011 by Routledge

Routledge
Taylor & Francis Group
711 Third Avenue
New York, NY 10017

Routledge
Taylor & Francis Group
2 Park Square, Milton Park
Abingdon, Oxon OX14 4RN

Abuse of Older Men has been co-published simultaneously as *Journal of Elder Abuse & Neglect*, Volume 19, Numbers 1/2 2007.

The development, preparation, and publication of this work has been undertaken with great care. However, the publisher, employees, editors, and agents of The Haworth Press and all imprints of The Haworth Press, including The Haworth Medical Press® and Pharmaceutical Products Press®, are not responsible for any errors contained herein or for consequences that may ensue from use of materials or information contained in this work. Opinions expressed by the author(s) are not necessarily those of The Haworth Press.

Library of Congress Cataloging-in-Publication Data

Abuse of older men/Jordan I. Kosberg, editor.
      p. cm.
   "Abuse of Older Men has been co-published simultaneously as Journal of elder abuse & neglect, volume 19, Numbers 1/2 2007."
     Includes bibliographical references and index.
     ISBN-13: 978-0-7890-3541-7 (hard cover : alk. paper)
     ISBN-13: 978-0-7890-3542-4 (soft cover : alk. paper)
1. Older men–Abuse of. 2. Older people–Abuse of. I. Kosberg, Jordan I., 1939- II. Journal of elder abuse & neglect.
HV6626.3.A273 2007
362.6--dc22
                                                          2007044630

ABOUT THE EDITOR

Jordan I. Kosberg, PhD, ACSW, has been The University of Alabama Endowed Chair of Social Work since 1999. He has taught at numerous universities in the United States and has been a Visiting Professor at Nankai University in Tianjin, China, at Hong Kong University, at City University of Hong Kong, and was the 2002 Visiting TOWER Fellow of the New Zealand Institute for Research on Ageing at Victoria University of Wellington. He is a Fellow of The Gerontological Society of America (GSA) and of the Association for Gerontology in Higher Education (AGHE). Dr. Kosberg is editor or co-editor of six books, and author or co-author of 25 book chapters and over 100 journal articles. Dr. Kosberg was recently the Co-Principal Investigator for two research projects on family caregiving funded by the National Institute on Aging and the Agency for Healthcare Research and Quality. He is former Board Member for the Association for Gerontology in Higher Education-Social Work (AGE-SW) and was awarded the Association's Career Achievement Award in 2000. He had been a member of the Board of Directors (representing the U.S.A. Region) for the International Network for the Prevention of Elder Abuse (a U.N. designated NGO).

Abuse
of Older Men

CONTENTS

Introduction   1
    Jordan I. Kosberg, PhD, ACSW

Intimate Partner Abuse of Older Men:
    Considerations for the Assessment of Risk   7
    Kim A. Reeves, MA
    Sarah L. Desmarais, MA
    Tonia L. Nicholls, PhD
    Kevin S. Douglas, LLB, PhD

From Behind the Shadows: A Profile of the Sexual Abuse
    of Older Men Residing in Nursing Homes   29
    Pamela B. Teaster, PhD
    Holly Ramsey-Klawsnik, PhD
    Marta S. Mendiondo, PhD
    Erin Abner, MPH
    Kara Cecil, BS
    Mary Tooms, BS

Detection and Prevalence of Abuse of Older Males:
   Perspectives from Family Practice   47
     Mark J. Yaffe, MD, MClSc
     Deborah Weiss, MSc
     Christina Wolfson, PhD
     Maxine Lithwick, MSW

Osteoporosis: An Invisible, Undertreated,
   and Neglected Disease of Elderly Men   61
     Marilyn L. Haas, PhD, RN, CNS, ANP-C
     Katen Moore, MSN, APRN, BC, AOCN®

Fractured Relationships and the Potential
   for Abuse of Older Men   75
     Dorothy C. Stratton, MSW, ACSW
     Alinde J. Moore, PhD

Notes on Newspaper Accounts of Male Elder Abuse   99
     R. L. McNeely, PhD, JD
     Philip W. Cook, BS

Identifying and Working with Older Male Victims
   of Abuse in England   109
     Jacki Pritchard, MA

Gendered Policies and Practices
   that Increase Older Men's Risk
   of Elder Mistreatment   129
     Edward H. Thompson Jr., PhD
     William Buxton, BA
     P. Casey Gough, BA
     Cara Wahle, BA

Intervention with Abused Older Males:
   Conceptual and Clinical Perspectives   153
     Lenard W. Kaye, DSW, PhD
     Diane Kay, MSW
     Jennifer A. Crittenden, MSW

Abuse of Elderly Male Clients: Efforts and Experiences
   in Rural and Urban Adult Protective Services   173
    Robert Blundo, PhD, LCSW
    Joseph Bullington, CSM

Index   193

Introduction

Jordan I. Kosberg, PhD, ACSW

This special addition of the *Journal of Elder Abuse & Neglect* (JEAN) focuses upon the abuse of older men. As such, it represents an extension of elder abuse literature that has, quite correctly, mainly focused upon the abuse of women who represent the majority of older persons. Yet, older men also are abused and, despite the likely under-reporting of many of these men, who is to say that their abuse should be of any less concern to us (whether as relatives, citizens, and/or professionals)?

So, too, this special issue of JEAN emanates out of the growing body of knowledge that suggests that there may be particular causes of, and consequences from, adversity faced by men, in general, and older men, in particular. The articles in this issue will offer reasons for believing that abused older men under-utilize community resources, although needed by them and available for them. Readers will come to understand that the failure of men to admit to having problems results, in part, from their denial, embarrassment, and stoicism. For similar reasons, older abused men can be reluctant to engage in help-seeking behavior. Finally, it will be suggested that older men may not be attracted to some resources, or have high dropout rates from others, as a result of the characteristics of the formal caregivers, clients or patients, the type of intervention, or the agency structures and procedures. Such possible deterrents for the use of needed community assistance for men are especially probable for older men who are abused, and it is imperative that those involved in the study, prevention, and intervention of elder abuse are sensitive to such possibilities with regard to older male abuse victims.

[Haworth co-indexing entry note]: "Introduction." Kosberg, Jordan I. Co-published simultaneously in *Journal of Elder Abuse & Neglect*™ (The Haworth Maltreatment & Trauma Press®, an imprint of The Haworth Press, Inc.) Vol. 19, No. 1/2, 2007, pp. 1-5; and: *Abuse of Older Men* (ed: Jordan I. Kosberg) The Haworth Maltreatment & Trauma Press®, an imprint of The Haworth Press, Inc., 2007, pp. 1-5. Single or multiple copies of this article are available for a fee from The Haworth Document Delivery Service [1-800-HAWORTH, 9:00 a.m. - 5:00 p.m. (EST). E-mail address: docdelivery@haworthpress.com].

Available online at http://jean.haworthpress.com
doi:10.1300/J084v19n01_01

One needs to be very cautious before saying that little has been published on any one topic. Relatively-speaking, elder abuse has been much less studied and discussed than have other forms of intra-family abuse. So, too, the abuse of older men has been much less studied and discussed than has the abuse of older women, and elder abuse continues to be considered mainly a problem affecting older women. Yet, there is an emerging body of literature on the abuse of older men. Although not referring solely to older men, in 1977-78, when Susan Steinmetz wrote of the "Battered Husband Syndrome," she brought awareness to the possibility that men, too, could be abused in domestic relationships. In 1997, Ted Koff discussed older men being "emotionally abused" within institutional settings where the majority of staff and residents were female and where activities were mainly "female oriented." Koff's work emphasized the problems resulting from incongruities in social settings for older men. In 1994, Edward Thompson, Jr. edited *Older Men's Lives,* which I consider to be among the most informative and influential texts on older men. While abusive behavior was not specifically covered in any of the chapters in Thompson's book, the material provided an excellent backdrop for work on older men, including the abuse of older men. Lenard Kaye and I edited, in 1997, *Elderly Men: Special Problems and Professional Challenges* that included a chapter on "The Victimization of Elderly Men" written by me and Stan Bowie. This chapter focused upon crime, institutional maltreatment, and elder abuse perpetrated against older men. The following year, 1998, I published in JEAN the article "The Abuse of Elderly Men" which provided the results of my exploration and conclusions about the problem.

Since the beginning of this decade, the literature on adversities faced by men (including older men) continued to increase. In 2001, Barbara Jo Brothers edited a special issue of the *Journal of Couples Therapy* that focused upon the abuse of men that included articles that focused upon abuse of men by their intimates, couples undergoing trauma-based transactions, and male partners of sexual abuse victims, but included no special attention to the abuse of older men. The articles in this special issue of the journal were simultaneously published by Haworth Press in *The Abuse of Men: Trauma Begets Trauma.* Also in 2001, Jacki Pritchard, from the United Kingdom, published perhaps the very first work that exclusively focused upon the abuse of older men, *Male Victims of Elder Abuse: Their Experiences and Needs.* This book was based upon her interviews with twelve older men who had experienced abuse. Thus, for well over a decade, there has been some attention given–either directly or indirectly–to the abuse of older men.

Yet, it is believed that the majority of material in this area has been rather general and in need to be extrapolated to older men. Moreover, elder abuse continues to be written and spoken about as mainly a problem perpetuated against women, and attention to the abuse of older men continues to be but an afterthought. A more focused approach highlighting elder abuse of men was believed needed and ultimately led to this special issue of JEAN.

The fact that abusers, in general, and elder abusers, in particular, are seen to be males also leads to a distorted and biased view against older men who could be victims. In 2002, I and Wiley Mangum wrote of "The Invisibility of Older Men in Gerontology," and suggested that aging and aged men have been largely ignored or downplayed in the literature and that their problems often have been ignored, misunderstood, or trivialized. In my article, "Meeting the Needs of Older Men: Challenges for Those in Helping Professions," that appeared in a 2005 special issue on older men published in the *Journal of Sociology and Social Welfare*, I discussed a number reasons for the lack of attention to the needs of older men, such as their smaller numbers, the belief that they enjoy a superior quality of life than women in their later years, sexist humor against older men (the "dirty old man"), the perception of such men as dependent and impaired, and other unfair and inaccurate stereotypes, among other overgeneralizations.

It is believed that this special issue of JEAN on abused older men will be helpful in making a case that elder abuse of men exists, and is invisible, under-studied, and under-treated. Perhaps underlying the need for making a case is a desire for gender equity in the focus on elder abuse and the concern for older persons–whether male or female and whether family members or clients and patients. Potential contributors to this special issue were either known to me by their work in the area of elder abuse or wrote in related areas. In the latter case, I appealed to them to refocus their efforts on the abuse of older men. It should be noted that contributors represent diverse backgrounds–law, health care, psychology, sociology, social work, criminology, among others. They are academics as well as practitioners.

The articles in this issue represent a broad range of concerns. A few articles identify abusive problems faced by some older men, such as sexual abuse (Pamela Teaster, Holly Ramsey-Klawsnick, Marta Mendiondo, Erin Abner, Kara Cecil, & Mary Toons), abuse by intimates (Kim Reeves, Sarah Desmarais, Tonia Nicholls, & Kevin Douglas), and benign neglect in the health care field (Marilyn Haas & Katen Moore). Several articles are written by those in the helping professions and are based upon either research findings and/or practice experiences from family medicine (Mark Yaffe, Deborah Weiss, Christina Wolfson, & Maxine Lithwick), adult protective services (Bob Blundo & Joseph Bullington), and social service departments (Jacki Pritchard). Attention to possible pre-determinants to abuse of older men is found in the article on consequences of poor relationships that had existed between older males and members of their family (Dorothy Stratton & Alinde Moore). Other articles discuss applied implications of knowledge for interventions with abused older men (Lenard Kaye, Diane Kay, & Jennifer Crittenden) and social policies that put older men at jeopardy (Edward Thompson, Jr., William Buxton, P. Casey Gough, & Cara Wahle). Finally, an article on newspaper reports on the abuse of older men (R.L. McNeely & Philip Cook) might offer a view of the "window" through which the public is made aware of this social problem. It should be noted that as a result of page limitations, among other considerations, there are two additional articles, one on the abuse of older male prisoners (Stan Stojkovic) and the other on the potential mistreatment of custodial grandfathers (Karen Bullock & Rebecca Thomas) that will be published in a subsequent issue of JEAN.

It is important to suggest that older men, as a group, are changing. It is believed that this group will become different from past and current cohorts who have represented more traditional male gendered values, attitudes, and behavior. Future cohorts of older men will, hopefully, be better socialized to support greater gender equitable norms in marriage, the family, and in society. It is also hoped that men will be less likely to engage in acts of omission and commission that have adversely affected members of their families and, thus, will be less likely to face the abuse of their children, wives, and partners in their later years. It is also hoped that boys will be less likely to be socialized to be aggressive, unemotional, and uncaring. It is too soon to know whether such changes in the nature of older men will result in the reduction or increase in their abuse.

Whether they are males or females, those who abuse older persons include those who would prey on older relatives or others out of anger, depression, incompetence, or financial or material gain and should be the focus of our concern in efforts to reduce the problem of elder abuse. Attention to the abuse of older men should be seen no different than attention to the abuse of older women. In the final analysis, the reasons for the abuse of older men or older women are more similar than different, including conditions that promote violence and abuse in society, and negatively characterizing older persons and other populations who are vulnerable, dependent, or perceived to be different.

Finally, it is hoped that this special edition of JEAN focusing upon the abuse of older men will help promote a general awareness of the fact that men, as well as women, are subject to elder abuse. Moreover, it is hoped that the professional community will acknowledge that older abused men may have different treatment needs and that the characteristics of both formal caregivers and health and social service resources need to consider older men's propensity for not admitting their adversities, seeking assistance, and being helped by different forms of interventions. The abuse of older men is no more important than is the abuse of older women; so, too, the abuse of older men is no less important than the abuse of older women.

REFERENCES

Brothers, B.J. (Ed.) (2001). *The Abuse of Men: Trauma Begets Trauma*. New York: The Haworth Press.

Koff, T.H. (1997). The institutionalization of elderly men. In J.I. Kosberg & L.W. Kaye (Eds.), *Elderly Men: Special Problems and Professional Challenges* (pp. 279-293). New York: Springer Publishing Company.

Kosberg, J.I. (2005). Meeting the needs of older men: Challenges for those in helping professions. *Journal of Sociology and Social Welfare, XXXII*(1): 9-31.

Kosberg, J.I. & Mangum, W.P. (2002). The invisibility of older men in gerontology. *Gerontology and Geriatric Education, 22*(4): 27-42.

Kosberg, J.I. & Bowie, S.L. (1997). The victimization of elderly men. In J.I. Kosberg & L.W. Kaye (Eds.), *Elderly Men: Special Problems and Professional Challenges* (pp. 216-229). New York: Springer Publishing Company.

Pritchard, J. (2001). *Male victims of elder abuse: Their experiences and needs*. London: Jessica Kingsley Publishers.

Steinmetz, S.K. (1977-78). The battered husband syndrome. *Victimology, 2*, 499.

Thompson, E.H., Jr. (Ed.)(1994). *Older Men's Lives*. Thousands Oaks, CA: Sage Publications.

doi:10.1300/J084v19n01_01

Intimate Partner Abuse of Older Men: Considerations for the Assessment of Risk

Kim A. Reeves, MA
Sarah L. Desmarais, MA
Tonia L. Nicholls, PhD
Kevin S. Douglas, LLB, PhD

Kim A. Reeves is a Graduate Student at Simon Fraser University, Department of Psychology, 8888 University Drive, Burnaby, British Columbia V5A 1S6 Canada (E-mail: kreeves@sfu.ca). Sarah L. Desmarais is a PhD Candidate at Simon Fraser University, Department of Psychology, 8888 University Drive, Burnaby, British Columbia V5A 1S6 Canada and Research Officer for the British Columbia Mental Health and Addiction Services (E-mail: sldesmar@sfu.ca). Tonia L. Nicholls is Senior Research Fellow at British Columbia Mental Health and Addiction Services, Forensic Psychiatric Hospital, 70 Colony Farm Road, Port Coquitlam, British Columbia, V3C 5X9, Canada and Adjunct Professor at Simon Fraser University, Department of Psychology, 8888 University Drive, Burnaby, British Columbia V5A 1S6 Canada (E-mail: tnicholls@forensic. bc.ca.). Kevin S. Douglas is Assistant Professor at Simon Fraser University, Department of Psychology, 8888 University Drive, Burnaby, British Columbia V5C 1S6 Canada (E-mail: douglask@sfu.ca).

For correspondence regarding this manuscript, please contact Kim Reeves (E-mail: kreeves@sfu.ca) at the above address.

The second and third authors wish to acknowledge the support of the Social Sciences and Humanities Research Council of Canada. The fourth author additionally is grateful to the Michael Smith Foundation for Health Research for their support.

[Haworth co-indexing entry note]: "Intimate Partner Abuse of Older Men: Considerations for the Assessment of Risk." Reeves, Kim A. et al. Co-published simultaneously in *Journal of Elder Abuse & Neglect*™ (The Haworth Maltreatment & Trauma Press®, an imprint of The Haworth Press, Inc.) Vol. 19, No. 1/2, 2007, pp. 7-27; and: *Abuse of Older Men* (ed: Jordan I. Kosberg) The Haworth Maltreatment & Trauma Press®, an imprint of The Haworth Press, Inc., 2007, pp. 7-27. Single or multiple copies of this article are available for a fee from The Haworth Document Delivery Service [1-800-HAWORTH, 9:00 a.m. - 5:00 p.m. (EST). E-mail address: docdelivery@haworthpress.com].

Available online at http://jean.haworthpress.com
doi:10.1300/J084v19n01_02

SUMMARY. Intimate partner abuse among older persons, though less common than among the general population, is a significant concern. Drawing from the intimate partner abuse and elder abuse literatures, this paper presents considerations for the assessment of risk for intimate partner abuse perpetrated against older men, with reference to the prevalent gendered view of abuse between intimate partners. Potential victim and perpetrator risk factors specific to this context are discussed and existing risk assessment tools are introduced. Implications and future research directions are discussed with regard to the application of risk assessment technology to this context. doi:10.1300/J084v19n01_02 *[Article copies available for a fee from The Haworth Document Delivery Service: 1-800-HAWORTH. E-mail address: <docdelivery@haworthpress.com> Website: <http://www.HaworthPress.com> © 2007 by The Haworth Press, Inc. All rights reserved.]*

KEYWORDS. Intimate partner abuse, risk assessment, elder abuse, gender bias, risk factors, vulnerability factors

INTRODUCTION

Although older adults are less likely to be the victims of violent crimes (e.g., theft, rape) relative to other demographic groups, many are at risk to be victimized by their family, friends, and caretakers through elder abuse (e.g., Backman, Dillaway, & Lachs, 1998). Next to adult children, the majority of elder abuse is perpetrated by spouses, and therefore can be considered intimate partner abuse (IPA) (National Center on Elder Abuse [NCEA], 1998). Though IPA in older populations is not as common as in younger populations, it is a significant concern in older persons because of the potential vulnerability due to the physical frailty and isolation of this population (Krug et al., 2002). Although older men are victims of IPA (as are younger men), this reality often is overlooked within the dominant feminist IPA perspective that considers men to be perpetrators, and women to be victims (Dutton & Nicholls, 2005). Increasingly being used with female victims in the general population, risk assessment instruments may have an important role to play in the prevention and management of IPA among older persons, and specifically among older men.

In this paper, we first introduce IPA among older adults generally and then specifically for older men, with reference to the prevalent "gendered" view of IPA. Historically, only men were recognized as perpetrators of

IPA but now it is well established that, overall, women are as likely to abuse their partners (for a review see Hamel & Nicholls, 2007). Second, we discuss victim and perpetrator risk factors and introduce existing risk assessment instruments for IPA as well as for elder abuse generally. Third, we consider the appropriateness of these risk assessment measures and special considerations that should be taken into account by mental health professionals working with this population. Lastly, we discuss implications and propose future research directions.

Existing risk assessment instruments assess for *violence*, not acts of omission such as neglect. Thus, to present considerations for the assessment of risk for IPA in older men, a definition of IPA that closely matches the definition of violence used by risk assessment instruments is warranted. As such, we will focus on *severe* IPA in this paper. The definition of violence used in the *Historical, Clinical, Risk Management–20* (HCR-20; Webster, Douglas, Eaves, & Hart, 1997), a structured professional judgment risk assessment scheme, defines violence as an "actual, attempted, or threatened harm to a person or persons" (p. 24). We also draw from the wider IPA literature in which IPA is defined as a pattern of physical, psychological, and/or sexual abuse by an intimate partner (Tjaden & Thoennes, 2000). For the present paper, we adapt both the HCR-20 general violence definition and the IPA definition to define IPA of older men as *an act or acts of commission by an intimate partner that causes harm to an older man (age 60 years and older), and which falls into one of the following categories: physical, psychological, or sexual.*

We adopt this definition with a few issues in mind. First, we refrain from using the term "elderly" because of its potentially pejorative connotation (American Psychological Association, 2001). Second, defining the age range for this cohort is difficult. Most people in the Western world consider old age to coincide with retirement age (~60 to 65 years; Krug et al., 2006). Also, most people can apply for Medicare in the US at the age of 65 (Centers for Medicare and Medicare Services, 2005) and the majority of state legislation defines an "older person" as either over the age of 60 or 65 years of age (American Bar Association Commission on Law and Aging, 2006). Third, intimate partner is defined as a dating partner, common-law partner, or spouse in alignment with the broader IPA literature (e.g., Tjaden & Thoennes, 2000). Financial abuse, although a category of elder abuse, will not be explored as such abuse is more likely to be perpetrated by an adult child than an intimate partner (e.g., NCEA, 1998) and is beyond the scope of the present paper.

INTIMATE PARTNER ABUSE (IPA)

Gender Bias

There is increasing evidence to contradict the notion that only men can be violent toward their romantic partners (Archer, 2000). However, feminist theories of power and control have continued to dominate the field of IPA, asserting that female violence is *always* in response to initial provocation by the male partner, and that women *always* suffer more se-rious injuries than men (for a full review of feminist theory and IPA see Dutton & Nicholls, 2005). The presumption that *all* men are potential abus-ers and women the *only* victims of IPA permeates victim advocacy, the criminal justice professionals system, and society as a whole (Stewart & Maddren, 1997; Worthen & Varnado-Sullivan, 2005). Although research demonstrates that women act in self-defense (as do men) and generally suffer more serious injuries than men (e.g., Tjaden & Thoennes, 2000), denying that women also can be the aggressor has minimized the provi-sion of services to male victims and their children (Dutton & Nicholls). The experiences of older male victims of IPA have received even less attention.

IPA Among Older Persons

IPA of older adults, until recently, has been subsumed under the um-brella category of 'elder abuse' rather than being considered a unique con-struct (Straka & Montminy, 2006). This de-contextualization of IPA among older persons contributed to a focus on perpetrators and types of abuse that are unique to this population, such as neglect by adult children. Therefore, IPA of older persons becomes lost in between the broader IPA research focusing on younger victims, on the one hand, and elder abuse on the other (Straka & Montminy, 2006). It is important to explore re-search on IPA in older persons to help bridge the gap between the two literatures and call attention to an important but under-researched popu-lation. Because of the paucity of IPA literature focusing specifically on older persons, the prevalence rates of IPA have been distilled from the broader elder abuse literature. For example, in a stratified random sample of 2,000 community persons aged 65 years and older, Pillemer and Finkelhor (1988) found that 58% of the perpetrators of elder abuse were intimate partners (36% women; 22% men). In another study of 1,057 persons aged 65 years and older in Illinois who sought assistance from programs serving victims of abuse in domestic settings over a five year period (90% women), Lundy and Grossman (2004) found that 38% were abused by their current husband or ex-husband. It is unclear, however, whether the observed rates reflect a life-long cycle of abuse or late-life onset of violence (Mouton et al., 2004). In fact, the literature suggests three types of IPA among older adults: (1) IPA that has spanned the relationship and is similar to IPA among younger populations (e.g., Brandl & Horan, 2002), (2) IPA associated with increased dependency of one partner on the other and is similar to elder abuse more broadly (e.g., Pillemer, 1985), and (3) a unique form of IPA associated with the onset of age-related cognitive impairments in the perpetrator (e.g., Paveza et al., 1992).

Older Men as Victims of IPA

Prevalence rates for IPA perpetrated against older men are currently unknown. Pillemer and Finkelhor (1988) reported greater rates of wife-to-husband than husband-to-wife abuse, but this finding is not replicated in the majority of studies. Research in the wider IPA context has found that men and women are more equal in their rates of perpetration than previously reported. In a meta-analysis of physical aggression in heterosexual partners, Archer (2000) found that women are equally likely or more likely to perpetrate IPA than men and less serious IPA in particular (e.g., slapping as opposed to choking). In addition, results indicated that although women aggress more frequently, they are also injured more often than men (62% of partners reporting injuries were women). These findings are relatively consistent across dating, cohabitating, and marital relationships in community samples (Dutton, Nicholls, & Spidel, 2005).

Given the comparable rates of male and female perpetrated IPA among the general population, it is important to explore the issue of IPA against older men. Part of this exploration should include a focus on prevention and management strategies. Risk assessment instruments, and structured professional judgment schemes specifically (to be defined and reviewed in more detail later in this paper), comprise factors identified in empirical and theoretical literature, as well as best practices, to guide the assessment of risk for future IPA and the development of risk management strategies. The following two sections review the literature on risk factors for the victimization and perpetration of IPA against older men.

VICTIM RISK FACTORS

What little is known regarding IPA victimization in older men has been learned primarily, and almost incidentally, from studies intended to examine IPA perpetrated against older women or abuse of older persons more generally. For example, using the *National Violence Against Women Survey*, Jasinski and Dietz (2003) examined physical abuse and stalking victimization among a sample of adults aged 55 years and older ($N =$ 3,622). Although the authors concluded that women were significantly more likely than men to be physically assaulted, the actual difference is arguably small (men = 0.6%; women = 1.9%). Importantly, victims of IPA, whether female or male, young or old, are a heterogeneous group. For example, research demonstrates that women who are in violent relationships are not demonstrably atypical of women in the general population, and efforts to identify a single IPA victim typology have failed (for a review see Rhodes & McKenzie, 1998). Nonetheless, extrapolating from the above-mentioned literatures, we review here risk factors which may be particularly relevant to IPA victimization in older men, including fear, living situation, social isolation, and cognitive and physical impairments.

Fear

Often referenced in the IPA literature, many authors suggest that fear is of particular importance to older adult victims (for review see Chu & Kraus, 2004). Specifically, research has documented an increased fear of crime and victimization in older persons, which has been found to be associated with immobility and decreased levels of functioning (e.g., Hennen & Knudten, 2001). This fear may in turn be coupled with fears associated with the reporting of such victimization. For example, experiences with the criminal justice system may actually heighten fear among older victims, as a result of difficulty in dealing with novel situations, concerns regarding perpetrator retaliation, and feelings of revictimization and intimidation in the face of questioning strategies which seek to discredit their testimony or allegations (Hirschel & Rubin, 1982). Such fears may be heightened in older men compared to women given that allegations of male victimization are both less likely to be reported in the first place and, if reported, generally are taken less seriously by professionals than IPA reports by women (Dutton & Nicholls, 2005).

Living Situation

The stress and demands associated with caregiving also are frequently discussed in the elder abuse literature (e.g., Lundy & Grossman, 2004). Research demonstrates that risk of victimization is heightened when the caregiver and care recipient co-reside, in that stress and conflict are difficult to avoid (e.g., George & Gwyther, 1986). For example, in their analyses of quantitative and qualitative data from 236 family caregivers of persons living with dementia, Pillemer and Suitor (1992) found that a shared living situation, in addition to physical aggression and disruptive behaviors by the care recipient, was predictive of violent feelings and aggression on the part of caregivers. Given that older women are more likely to outlive their spouses and live alone compared to older men, who tend to live with a spouse or partner (Lundy & Grossman), living situation may be especially pertinent to the victimization of older men.

Social Isolation

Characteristic of IPA, social isolation, "a lack of social interaction" (Hughes & Gove, 1981, p. 50), may contribute to a failure to identify incidents of IPA as abuse, thereby preventing the reporting of such incidents. Without external referencing, there is an increased likelihood that IPA will be viewed as normal behavior (e.g., Phillips, Torres de Ardon, & Briones, 2000). Victims of IPA may be socially isolated as a result of perpetrator attempts to prevent contact with others. Older adults are particularly likely to experience social isolation due to circumstances associated with their age (e.g., few remaining living friends and/or family) or physical health (e.g., inability to leave their residence unaided). Even if victims are not isolated, family and friends may not support attempts to seek help or end the relationship for reasons associated with generational differences in beliefs about normative spousal behaviors (e.g., Ramsey-Klawsnik, 2003).

Cognitive Impairments

Cognitive impairments, such as confusion, are prominent among victims of elder abuse (including IPA); for example, the *National Elder Abuse Incidence Survey* (NCEA, 1998) reported that approximately 60% of elder abuse victims experienced confusion to varying degrees. Specific disorders, such as Alzheimer's and depression, also have been associated with increased risk for victimization (e.g., Anetzberger et al., 2000). In contrast, other research among patients with Alzheimer's disease failed to demonstrate that degree of impairment was a risk factor for abuse (e.g., Paveza et al., 1992), even though research suggests that violent victimization *is* more common among persons with mental disorders than those without mental disorders (e.g., Teplin, McClelland, & Abram, 2005). Importantly, as with psychopathology in younger IPA victim populations, it is unclear whether suffering such a disorder increases the likelihood that older men will be abused or whether victims become depressed or impaired as a consequence.

Physical Impairments

Physical health problems and frailty also may be associated with IPA victimization among older men. Pillemer and Finkelhor (1988) found that older adults in poor health were three to four times more likely to be victims of elder abuse than those in good health. However, beyond a certain threshold, further degree of physical and/or cognitive impairment does not appear to moderate level of risk (Cooney, Howard, & Lawlor, 2006); that is, it is the presence, and not the degree, of such impairments which increases risk. Further, physical disabilities, such as confinement to a wheelchair, may increase the effect and/or importance of previously discussed victim characteristics, such as isolation. Importantly, frailty associated with old age can increase the prevalence and seriousness of injury resulting from physical aggression (e.g., Chu & Kraus, 2004).

In sum, consistent with early attempts to identify the psychopathology of abused women, empirical evidence suggests that there is no single typology of an older male victim of IPA. However, research has identified several factors or characteristics that are associated with IPA victimization and which may be useful in identifying at risk individuals. As we noted above, research findings examining IPA in older adults often are consistent with the general spousal assault and dating abuse literatures suggesting similar perpetrator and victim risk factors might be relevant to risk assessment and abuse prevention strategies.

PERPETRATOR RISK FACTORS

There is increasing evidence that IPA among older persons reflects many of the same dynamics that have been present throughout the relationship as opposed to dynamics that developed with older age, with age-specific psychopathology as the exception (e.g., Alzheimer's). As such, there are likely many perpetrator risk factors common to IPA across the lifespan (e.g., Wilke & Vinton, 2005). The following is a review of risk factors which may be particularly relevant to the context of IPA among older men, including mental illness, cognitive impairments, and relationship dependency. Substance abuse, although not unique to this context, is included to draw attention to this emerging and under recognized problem.

Mental Illness and Cognitive Impairments

The relationship between mental illness and cognitive impairments and the perpetration of aggressive and violent behavior among older adults is well documented (e.g., Miller et al., 2006). Dementia and depression are two commonly cited disorders of particular importance to the older population, primarily because of their association with Alzheimer's disease, but also as psychiatric illnesses in and of themselves.

In addition to the agitation and aggression symptomatic of the disorder (e.g., Mirakhur, Craig, Hart, McIlroy, & Passmore, 2004), one of the common delusions among individuals suffering from dementia is of spousal infidelity (Leroi, Voulgari, Breitner, & Lyketsos, 2003; Tsai, Hwang, Yang, & Liu, 1997). Although some research suggests that women suffering from Alzheimer's disease are at higher risk for delusions generally than are men (Leroi et al., 1998), this particular category of delusions appears to affect older men and women at comparable rates (e.g., Tsai et al.). Long recognized as a motive for violence, the implications of such *delusional jealousy* can be serious; for example, Tsai et al. found that many patients included in their study acted on these beliefs, including attempts at social isolation, as well as verbal and physical abuse.

There is also a body of research demonstrating depression manifesting as agitation and aggression among older persons. Although research findings regarding whether the prevalence of depression increases or decreases with age are mixed (e.g., Kessler, Foster, Webster, & House, 1992; Streiner, Cairney, & Veldhuizen, 2006), depressive symptomatology is commonly associated with dementia in aged populations, as noted earlier. Whatever the etiology, such symptoms appear to accompany both physical and verbal aggression in this context, and research suggests that cognitive impairments and depression are precursors to agitation which in turn is expressed through overt aggression (Cohen-Mansfield, Marx, & Werner, 1992).

Substance Abuse

Substance abuse disorders are arguably under diagnosed in older persons, for reasons including ageism (e.g., healthcare and mental health professionals are less likely to screen for drug or alcohol abuse in this population), poor identification of symptoms, and a lack of knowledge about assessment techniques (e.g., Knauer, 2003). One study of 549 primary care patients aged 65 years and older who reported drinking one or more alcoholic beverages in the past 12 months labeled 11% of participants as harmful drinkers (i.e., associated with the likely presence of alcohol-related problems) and 35% as hazardous drinkers (i.e., associated with complications in medical diagnosis and treatment, posing risks for medical/psychosocial problems, and precipitating adverse drug reactions) (Fink et al., 2002). Specifically, the existing research on elder abuse, as well as the IPA literature, demonstrates that drug and/or alcohol use increases the likelihood of abuse perpetration, by both male and female partners (e.g., Bradshaw & Spencer, 1999; Stuart, Moore, Ramsey, & Kahler, 2003). Substance abuse may serve to reduce perpetrator inhibitions and increase rationalization of the behavior (*cf.* Fals-Stewart & Kennedy, 2005).

Relationship Dependency

In contrast to the popular belief that older victims of IPA are dependent on their abuser, considerable research suggests that the opposite is true: it is the dependent partner, acting in response to feelings of powerlessness in the relationship, who is more likely to be the abuser (e.g., Pillemer, 1985). Consistent with the general IPA literature, power (or perhaps more appropriately, feelings of powerlessness and dependence on the victim for financial assistance, housing, transportation, or care) may be important in the perpetration of IPA against older men (e.g., Brownell, Berman, & Salamone, 1989). Under the *power and control* model of IPA, the "abusive behavior is used by the abuser in order to gain and maintain power and control in the relationship" (Kernsmith, 2005, p. 174; see also Johnson, 2001). Some research has demonstrated that men are more likely to abuse power and control (Coker et al., 2002), whereas women report using violence in response to prior abuse (Kernsmith). Importantly, however, reviews suggest that women's motives for perpetrating IPA are highly similar to those of men (Dutton & Nicholls, 2005). To demonstrate, women in the Kernsmith study *did* report motivations frequently associated with personal control.

As our review suggested for victim risk factors, there does not appear to be one typology of *the* IPA perpetrator, especially with regard to perpetration against older men. As mentioned earlier in this section, only recently has the perpetration of IPA by women against men been acknowledged, and the research and theoretical literature is still in its infancy. Importantly, readers are reminded that our discussion represents only a summary of characteristics we propose might be especially pertinent in or unique to this context and is not meant to be seen as an exhaustive review. Risk assessment theory and the broader literature on risk factors for spousal assault and existing technologies are likely to inform this emerging field of research and important branch of clinical practice.

RISK ASSESSMENT

We have delineated several potentially important risk factors for IPA among older men. Although this is important in terms of understanding its phenomenology, it does not provide specific guidance to clinicians and other decision-makers about how to assess for the risk for such abuse. Early detection and/or prevention of IPA among older adults will not only improve quality of life, but also will reduce their reliance on the health care system (Brandl & Horan, 2002). In this section, we provide a brief overview of risk assessment decision-making approaches that have been used in other contexts to estimate a person's risk for perpetrating violence to others.

More than 50 years ago, Paul Meehl (1954) drew an important distinction between two types of prediction–clinical and actuarial. Since that time, researchers have concluded that unstructured clinical prediction is not sufficiently reliable or valid to form the basis of defensible predictions (or estimates) about the likelihood of a future event (e.g., Grove, Zald, Lebow, Snitz, & Nelson, 2000). Two major alternatives have been developed in response, and underpin the development of contemporary violence risk assessment theory and instruments. The first, the *actuarial* approach, has a long history in psychology and related disciplines, and can be defined as "a formal method, [that] uses an equation, a formula . . . to arrive at a probability or expected value, of some outcome" (Grove & Meehl, 1996, p. 294). Meta-analytic research suggests that actuarial prediction is more accurate than unstructured clinical prediction in approximately 50% of research studies (Grove et al., 2000).

Despite these advantages, criticism has been directed toward a strict actuarial approach in the violence risk assessment field (Douglas & Kropp, 2002) for reasons including the general absence of dynamic (i.e., changeable) risk factors that represent promising risk reduction and treatment opportunities (Douglas & Skeem, 2005) and limited evidence for their application beyond development samples (Hart, 1998). In response to these criticisms, *structured professional judgment* (SPJ) schemes have been developed for the assessment of violence risk (e.g., Webster et al., 1997). The SPJ model structures decisions by specifying which factors should be considered in every risk assessment, providing explicit operational definitions and coding procedures for each item, providing guidance for the making of final decisions, and providing professional manuals that specify user qualifications, assessment methods, and general information about risk assessment for the type of violence under consideration. Research supports the validity of these instruments in predicting violence (e.g., Douglas, Yeomans, & Boer, 2005).

Risk Assessment in IPA

Spousal Assault Instruments. In comparison to considerable progress in the general risk assessment field, the domestic violence field has lagged behind in this important effort to bridge science and practice. In recent years, a selection of IPA risk assessment instruments have been developed, several of which are the focus of current validation efforts (for reviews see Dutton & Kropp, 2000; Nicholls et al., 2007). Many of the risk factors relevant to general offending are common to partner abuse and there is also good consensus between the different domestic violence risk assessment schemes. A comprehensive review of these instruments is beyond the scope of this paper. We provide a select discussion of risk assessment schemes that have been validated in published research with female victims of abuse, the Danger Assessment (Campbell, 1995), the Spousal Assault Risk Assessment guide (Kropp et al., 1999), and the Ontario Domestic Assault Risk Assessment. To our knowledge none of these instruments have been validated with male victims or older adult victims.

The *Danger Assessment* (DA, Campbell, 1986, 1995, 2006) is one of the earliest and most widely studied spousal assault instruments. It is unique from other measures we discuss, in that its purpose is to help victims evaluate the likelihood that their partner presents a risk of *homicide*, and not evaluate risk of recidivistic partner abuse. The assessment is intended to be completed by a nurse and the woman together, and it is expected that it will increase women's self-care agency (i.e., ability to safety plan; Campbell, 1986). The items on the DA initially were identified from retrospective research studies of female victims of serious IPA and victims of homicide (Campbell). The measure was then discussed with battered women, shelter workers, law enforcement officials, and other experts (Campbell). The DA has been the focus of several validation studies and recently was revised to reflect findings from a multi-site case control study of femicide (Campbell). The literature suggests that although several of the items might be relevant to an assessment of a female perpetrator's risk of killing their male partner (e.g., access to weapons–women use weapons to even the differential strength of men and women), others are unlikely to be relevant (e.g., a history of choking–women are less likely than men to choke their partners) or are clearly gender specific (e.g., prior abuse during pregnancy).

The *Spousal Assault Risk Assessment* guide (SARA; Kropp, Hart, Webster, & Eaves, 1999) is a 20-item SPJ instrument designed to assess adult men for risk of abuse against female intimate partners. Items on the SARA were identified primarily from the scientific and professional literatures on characteristics of assaultive men and the predictors of violent crime, as described in the discussion of SPJ instruments above. Part 1 consists of 10 general violence risk factors (e.g., past assault of family members, past assault of strangers or acquaintances) and Part 2 consists of 10 partner violence risk factors (e.g., past physical assault, past sexual assault, extreme minimization/denial, and attitudes that support or condone spousal assault). Using SPJ, assessors use the item descriptions to form a clinical evaluation of future spouse abuse (i.e., low, moderate or high). The SARA has been evaluated in several studies (e.g., Grann & Wedin, 2002; Hilton et al., 2004; Kropp & Hart, 2000; Williams & Houghton, 2002); however, none speaks to its relevance to IPA among older adults or the perpetration of IPA by women.

The *Ontario Domestic Assault Risk Assessment* (ODARA; Hilton et al., 2004) is an actuarial instrument that assesses the likelihood that a man will assault his female domestic partner again and determines how his risk compares with that of other male intimate assaulters. Using multiple regression techniques, the authors of the ODARA examined just less than 600 cases of IPA and identified 13 yes/no questions most predictive of future *male* perpetrated *heterosexual* partner abuse. The questions addressed include variables relevant to the accused man's history of violence and antisocial behavior (e.g., police record for domestic assault, substance abuse), details of the most recent assault (e.g., physical confinement), and the victim's personal circumstances (e.g., barriers to support). This instrument was developed and has been tested in cases involving male-to-female partner assaults among current or former co-habiting or marital relationships. As a result, its relevance to other abusive relationships such as female perpetrated aggression against male partners, abuse in older adults, gay and lesbian relationships, or among dating partners is not yet known. Many of the ODARA items (and items on the other measures) are common to the general violence risk assessment field and are likely to be robust predictors of IPA perpetration independent of perpetrator and victim gender (e.g., Hilton et al., 2004).

Risk Assessment in Elder Abuse

Instruments that exist for the assessment of elder abuse can be divided into two categories: (1) instruments that screen for elder abuse (for review see Fulmer, Guadagno, Bitondo-Dyer, & Connolly, 2004) and (2) instruments that assess future risk of elder abuse (Goodrich, 1997). The former category of instruments was developed to aid detection, assessment, and intervention in cases of elder abuse (Ansell & Breckman, 1988). In a study of instruments used by Adult Protective Services (APS) programs, the majority were classified as screening measures or diagnostic measures and none were prognostic (identifying predictors of outcome) (Johnson, 1989). However, the settings for conducting risk assessments for IPA in older men do not completely overlap with settings for IPA risk assessments. These men are more likely to come in contact with health professionals than with the criminal justice system. Therefore, screening measures are vital in the development of intervention strategies and management plans for both the victim and the perpetrator (Fulmer et al.).

Instruments in the latter category were developed to evaluate risk for the perpetration of elder abuse (Goodrich, 1997). According to Anetzberger (2001), none of the elder abuse screening instruments or referral protocols specifically address IPA. To address this need, Anetzberger and colleagues developed *Screening Tools and Referral Protocol for Stopping Abuse Against Older Ohioans: A Guide for Service Providers* (STRP; Bass, Anetzberger, Ejaz, & Nagpaul, 2001). It includes the *Risk of Abuse Tool*, a one-page checklist of 28 risk factors both for the victim and perpetrator that were identified in the literature as being associated with IPA among older adults. Five "extended" tools are included to aid in assessing the presence or absence of the risk factors. There are currently no published reliability or validity data on the STRP, nor is it clear how

IPA is incorporated into the *Risk of Abuse Tool itself, or if it is only part of the discussion of elder abuse in the main portion of the protocol.*

Goodrich (1997) conducted a survey of state APS programs to examine their documentation systems, the use of risk assessment, and the program outcome measures. Results demonstrated that 18 states used risk assessments tools which described the client's current level of risk for future elder abuse based on at least one of the following categories: (1) victim risk factors, (2) environmental risk factors (e.g., structural soundness of the house), (3) support services, (4) current and historical abuse factors (e.g., severity and escalation of types of abuse), and (5) perpetrator risk factors. No information was available regarding whether these measures were standardized across states, or whether the tools had been validated. However, the author did comment that states tend not to have the resources to develop reliable and valid risk assessment measures.

Assessment of Risk for IPA Among Older Men

Elder abuse instruments are unclear in their treatment of IPA. Similarly, current spousal assault risk assessment instruments are ambiguous in their relevance to female perpetration and male victimization. In addition, current iterations of spousal assault risk assessment instruments either do not include victim risk factors or do not consider a wide range of victim risk factors or what are sometimes referred to as victim vulnerability factors. Further, some of the risk factors specific to IPA among the older population are not included in existing spousal assault instruments: (1) age-associated cognitive impairments, (2) fear, (3) living situation, (4) physical impairments, and (5) dependency. Some of these factors may be assessed indirectly through consideration of the perpetrator's controlling behaviors (dependency), employment and financial difficulties (dependency), severe mental illness (cognitive impairments), and separation from partner (living situation). However, an important limitation of the spousal assault instruments is that all were developed for the case of male violence perpetrated against a female intimate partner. As such, existing tools should be used with caution, if at all, in the assessment of cases involving male victimization. Until risk factors for female perpetration are established or the predictive validity of existing instruments is examined in such cases, the task of preventing and managing IPA of men remains especially challenging.

IMPLICATIONS AND RESEARCH DIRECTIONS

The limitations noted above lead to a consideration of future directions in the assessment of IPA among older men. The infancy of the research and literature on the perpetration of IPA by women against men, and even more so among the older population (this is also true of gay and lesbian IPA), has been a recurring theme in this paper. There *have* been considerable advances in the assessment and management of IPA as well as elder abuse; however, considerable empirical research is still needed. For instance, there is insufficient evidence (e.g., from cross-validation and prospective studies with large samples) to suggest an instrument that might be considered the "gold standard" in clinical practice among the general population, let alone among the older population. Further, as emphasized throughout this paper, relative to the literature examining risk factors for male-perpetrated abuse, there is limited research examining which variables are most predictive of women's risk to abuse intimate partners. Preliminary findings suggest that many risk factors (such as items in the measures discussed above) are likely relevant regardless of the perpetrators' gender (e.g., Dutton et al., 2005). Importantly, however, there may be factors specific to the context of such behavior among older persons that require additional consideration.

A related issue is what to do once such a risk has been identified. Unfortunately, empirical evidence demonstrating the efficacy of interventions with perpetrators is lacking. Research suggests that treatment programs for abusive men in the health sector have had minimal effects on recidivism. For example, a meta-analysis of treatment outcome studies demonstrated very small effect sizes for interventions with male batterers (Babcock, Green, & Robie, 2004). Correspondingly, Kropp and Hart (2000) stated that IPA perpetrators, even those who have participated in treatment, have the highest rate of recidivism of all violent offenders. Some studies suggest that treatment programs for abusers actually may increase the victim's risk because victims report returning to the relationship *because of* the perpetrator's participation in treatment (Babcock & Steiner, 1999). Additionally, many jurisdictions in North America have implemented mandatory arrest policies and treatment programs for perpetrators of IPA (e.g., Babcock & Steiner, 1999; Kropp & Hart). Are these policies and programs extended to IPA in the context of older persons? Again, empirical research must examine the appropriateness of existing interventions, policies, and programs for female perpetrators of IPA, and among the older population specifically.

In conclusion, research on issues in IPA in older persons and female perpetrators is lagging behind the needs of clinical practice. The perpetuation of the gender bias across age groups is hindering the progress of assessment and intervention strategies and therefore not providing needed services for older men who are victims of IPA.

REFERENCES

American Bar Association Commission on Law and Aging, (2006). *Analysis of state adult protective services laws.* Retrieved November 30, 2006 from http://www.elderabusecenter.org/default.cfm?p=statelawsanalysis.cfm

American Psychological Association. (2001). Publication manual of the *American Psychological Association* (5th ed.). *Washington, D.C.: Author.*

Anetzberger, G. J. (2001). Elder abuse identification and referral: The importance of screening tools and referral protocols. *Journal of Elder Abuse & Neglect, 13,* 3-22.

Anetzberger, G. J., Palmisano, B. R., Sanders, M., Bass, D., Dayton, C., Eckert, S. et al. (2000). A model intervention for elder abuse and dementia. *The Gerontologist, 40,* 492-497.

Ansell, P. & Breckman, R. (1988). *Elder mistreatment guidelines for health care professionals: Detection, assessment, and intervention.* New York: Mount Sinai/Victim Services Agency.

Archer, J. (2000). Sex differences in aggression between heterosexual partners: A meta-analytic review. *Psychological Bulletin, 126,* 651-680.

Babcock, J., & Steiner, R. (1999). The relationship between treatment, incarceration and recidivism on battering: A program evaluation of Seattle's Coordinated Community Response to domestic violence. *Journal of Family Psychology, 13,* 46-59.

Babcock, J. C., Green, C. E., & Robie, C. (2004). Does batterers' treatment work? A meta-analytic review of domestic violence treatment. *Clinical Psychology Review, 23,* 1023-1053.

Backman, R., Dillaway, H., & Lachs, M. S. (1998). Violence against the elderly: A comparative analysis of robbery and assault across age and gender groups. *Research on Aging, 20*(2), 183-198.

Bass, D. M., Anetzberger, G. J., Ejaz, F. K., & Nagpaul, K. (2001). Screening tools and referral protocol for stopping abuse against older Ohioans: A guide for service providers. *Journal of Elder Abuse & Neglect, 13,* 23-38.

Bradshaw, D., & Spencer, C. (1999). The role of alcohol in elder abuse cases. In J. Pritchard (Ed.), *Elder abuse: Good practices in prevention and intervention* (pp. 332-353). London: Kingsley.

Brandl, B., & Horan, D. L. (2002). Domestic violence later in life: An overview for health care providers. *Women and Health [Special issue], 35*(2/3), 41-54.

Brownell, P., Berman, J., & Salamone, A. (1989). Mental health and criminal justice issues among perpetrators of elder abuse. *Journal of Elder Abuse & Neglect, 11,* 81-94.

Campbell, J. C. (1986). Nursing assessment of risk of homicide for battered women. *Advances in Nursing Science, 3,* 67-85.

Campbell, J. C. (1995). Prediction of homicide of and by battered women. In J. C. Campbell (Ed.), *Assessing dangerousness: Violence by sexual offenders, batterers, and child abusers* (pp. 96-113). Thousand Oaks, CA: Sage.

Campbell, J. C. (2006). *The danger assessment.* Accessed January 4, 2006, from http://www.dangerassessment.com/WebApplication1/pages/product.aspx

Centers for Medicare and Medicare Services. (2005). *Overview.* Retrieved November 30, 2006 from http://www.cms.hhs.gov/MedicareGenInfo

Chu, L. D., & Kraus, J. F. (2004). Predicting fatal assault among the elderly using the National Incident-Based Reporting System Crime Data. *Homicide Studies, 8,* 71-95.

Cohen-Mansfield, J., Marx, M. S., & Werner, P. (1992). Agitation in elderly persons. An integrative report of findings in a nursing home. *International Psychogeriatrics, 4,* 221-240.

Coker, A. L., Davis, K. E., Arias, I., Desai, S., Sanderson, M., Brandt, H. M. et al. (2002). Physical and mental health effects of intimate partner violence for men and women. *American Journal of Preventative Medicine, 23,* 260-268.

Cooney, C., Howard, R., & Lawlor, B. (2006). Abuse of vulnerable people with dementia by their carers: Can we identify those most at risk? *International Journal of Geriatric Psychiatry, 21,* 564-571.

Douglas, K. S., & Kropp, P. R. (2002) A prevention-based paradigm for violence risk assessment: Clinical and research applications. *Criminal Justice & Behavior, 29,* 617-658.

Douglas, K. S., & Skeem, J. L. (2005). Violence risk assessment: Getting specific about being dynamic. *Psychology, Public Policy, and Law, 11,* 347-383.

Douglas, K. S., Yeomans, M., & Boer, D. P. (2005). Comparative validity analysis of multiple measures of violence risk in a general population sample of criminal offenders. *Criminal Justice and Behavior, 32,* 479-510.

Dutton, D. G., & Kropp, P. R. (2000). A review of domestic violence risk instruments. *Trauma, Violence and Abuse, 1,* 171-182.

Dutton, D. G., & Nicholls, T. L. (2005). The gender paradigm in domestic violence research and theory: Part 1–The conflict of theory and data. *Aggression and Violent Behavior, 10,* 680-714.

Dutton, D. G., Nicholls, T. L., & Spidel, A. (2005). Female perpetrators of intimate abuse. *Journal of Offender Rehabilitation, 41,* 1-31.

Fals-Stewart, W., & Kennedy, C. (2005). Addressing intimate partner violence in substance-abuse treatment. *Journal of Substance Abuse Treatment, 29,* 5-17.

Fink, A., Morton, S. A., Beck, J. C., Hays, R. D., Spritzer, K., Oishi, S. et al. (2002). Comparing the alcohol-related problems survey (ARPS) to traditional alcohol screening measures in elderly outpatients. *Archives of Gerontology and Geriatrics, 34,* 55-78.

Fulmer, T., Guadagno, L., Bitondo-Dyer, C., & Connolly, M. T. (2004). Progress in elder abuse screening and assessment instruments. *Journal of the American Geriatrics Society, 52,* 297-304.

George, L. K., & Gwyther, L. P. (1986). Caregiver well-being: A multidimensional examination of family caregivers of demented adults. *The Gerontologist, 26,* 253-259.

Goodrich, C. S. (1997). Results of a national survey of state protective services programs: Assessing risk and defining victim outcomes. *Journal of Elder Abuse & Neglect, 9,* 69-86.

Grann, M., & Wedin, I. (2002). Risk factors for recidivism among spousal assault and spousal homicide offenders. *Psychology, Crime, and Law, 8,* 5-23.

Grove, W. M., & Meehl, P. E. (1996). Comparative efficiency of informal (subjective, impressionistic) and formal (mechanical, algorithmic) prediction procedures: The clinical-statistical controversy. *Psychology, Public Policy, and Law, 2,* 293-323.

Grove, W. M., Zald, D. H., Lebow, B. S., Snitz, B. E., & Nelson, C. (2000). Clinical versus mechanical prediction: A meta-analysis. *Psychological Assessment, 12,* 19-30.

Hamel, J., & Nicholls, T. L. (2007). *Family therapy for domestic violence: A practitioner's guide to gender-inclusive research and treatment.* London: Springer.

Hart, S. D. (1998). The role of psychopathy in assessing risk for violence: Conceptual and methodological issues. *Legal & Criminological Psychology, 3,* 121-137.

Hart, S. D., Kropp, P. R., Laws, D. R., Klaver, J., Logan, C., & Watt, K. A. (2003). *The risk for sexual violence protocol.* Burnaby, BC: Simon Fraser University.

Hennen, J. R., & Knudten, R. D. (2001). A lifestyle analysis of the elderly: Perceptions of risk, fear, and vulnerability. *Illness, Crisis, & Loss, 9,* 190-208.

Hilton, N. Z., Harris, G. T., Rice, M. E., Lang, C., Cormier, C. A., & Lines, K. J. (2004). A brief actuarial assessment for the prediction of wife assault recidivism: The Ontario Domestic Assault Risk Assessment. *Psychological Assessment, 16,* 267-275.

Hughes, M., & Gove, W. R. (1981). Living alone, social integration, and mental health. *American Journal of Sociology, 87,* 48-74.

Jasinski, J. L., & Dietz, T. L. (2003). Domestic violence and stalking among older adults: An assessment of risk markers. *Journal of Elder Abuse & Neglect, 15,* 3-18.

Johnson, M .P. (2001). Conflict and control: Symmetry and asymmetry in domestic violence. In A. Booth & A. C. Crouter (Eds.), *Couples in conflict* (pp. 94-104). Mahwah, NJ: Lawrence Erlbaum Associates.

Johnson, T. F. (1989). Elder mistreatment identification instruments: Finding common ground. *Journal of Elder Abuse & Neglect, 1,* 15-37.

Kernsmith, P. (2005). Exerting power or striking back: A gendered comparison of motivations for domestic violence perpetration. *Violence and Victims, 20,* 173-185.

Kessler, R. C., Foster, C., Webster, P. S., & House, J. S. (1992). The relationship between age and depressive symptoms in two national surveys. *Psychology and Aging, 7,* 119-126.

Knauer, C. (2003). Geriatric alcohol abuse: A national epidemic. *Geriatric Nursing, 24,* 152-154.

Kropp, P. R., & Hart, S. D. (2000). The Spousal Assault Risk Assessment (SARA) guide: Reliability and validity in adult male offenders. *Law and Human Behavior, 24,* 101-118.

Kropp, P. R., Hart, S. D., Webster, C. D., & Eaves, D. (1999). *Manual for the Spousal Assault Risk Assessment Guide* (3rd ed.). Toronto, ON: Multi-Health Systems.

Krug, E., Dahlberg, L. L., Mercy, J. A., Zwi, A. B., & Lozano, R. (Eds.). (2002). *World report on violence and health.* Geneva: World Health Organization.

Leroi, I., Voulgari, A., Breitner, J. C. S., & Lyketsos, C. G. (2003). The epidemiology of psychosis in dementia. *American Journal of Geriatric Psychiatry, 11,* 83-91.

Lundy, M., & Grossman, S. F. (2004). Elder abuse: Spouse/intimate partner abuse and family violence among elders. *Journal of Elder Abuse & Neglect, 16*, 85-102.

Meehl, P. E. (1954). *Clinical versus statistical prediction*. Minneapolis, MN: University of Minnesota Press.

Miller, L. S., Lewis, M. S., Williamson, G. M., Lance, C. E., Dooley, W. K., Schulz, R. et al. (2006). Caregiver cognitive status and potentially harmful caregiver behavior. *Aging & Mental Health, 10*,125-133.

Mirakhur, A., Craig, D., Hart, D. J., McIlroy, S. P., & Passmore, A. P. (2004). Behavioural and psychological syndromes in Alzheimer's disease. *International Journal of Geriatric Psychiatry, 19*, 1035-1039.

Mouton, C. P., Rodabough, R. J., Rovi, S. L. D., Hunt, J. L., Talamantes, M. A., Brzyski, R. G. et al. (2004). Prevalence and 3-year incidence of abuse among postmenopausal women. *American Journal of Public Health, 94*, 604-612.

National Center on Elder Abuse. (1998). *The national elder abuse incidence study: Final report*. Washington, D.C.: American Public Health Services Association.

Nicholls, T. L., Desmarais, S. L., Douglas, K. S., & Kropp, P. R. (2007). Assessment of high risk perpetrators of intimate partner abuse. In J. Hamel & T. L. Nicholls (Eds.), *Family therapy for domestic violence: A practitioner's guide to gender-inclusive research and treatment* (pp. 275-301). London: Springer.

Paveza, G. J., Cohen, D., Eisdorfer, C., Freels, S., Semla, T., Ashford, J. W. et al. (1992). Severe family violence and Alzheimer's disease: Prevalence and risk factors. *Gerontologist, 32*, 493-497.

Phillips, L., Torres de Ardon, E., & Briones, G. (2000). Abuse of female caregivers by care recipients: Another form of elder abuse. *Journal of Elder Abuse & Neglect, 12*, 123-144.

Pillemer, K. (1985). The dangers of dependency: New findings on domestic violence against the elderly. *Social Problems, 33*, 146-158.

Pillemer, K., & Finkelhor, D. (1988). The prevalence of elder abuse: A random sample survey. *Gerontologist, 28*, 51-57.

Pillemer, K., & Finkelhor, D. (1989). Causes of elder abuse: Caregiver stress versus problem relatives. *American Journal of Orthopsychiatry, 59*, 179-187.

Pillemer, K., & Suitor, J. J. (1992). Violence and violent feelings: What causes them among family caregivers? *Journals of Gerontology, 47*, S165-S172.

Ramsey-Klawsnik, H. (2003). Elder sexual abuse within the family. *Journal of Elder Abuse & Neglect, 15*, 43-58.

Rhodes, N. R., & McKenzie, E. B. (1998). Why do battered women stay?: Three decades of research. *Aggression and Violent Behavior, 3*, 391-406.

Stewart, A., & Maddren, K. (1997). Police officers' judgements of blame in family violence: The impact of gender and alcohol. *Sex Roles, 37*, 921-933.

Straka, S. M., & Montminy, L. (2006). Responding to the needs of older women experiencing domestic violence. *Violence Against Women, 12*, 251-267.

Streiner, D. L., Cairney, J., & Veldhuizen, S. (2006). The epidemiology of psychological problems in the elderly. *Canadian Journal of Psychiatry, 51*, 185-191.

Stuart, G. L., Moore, T. M., Ramsey, S. E., & Kahler, C. W. (2003). Relationship aggression and substance use among women court-referred to domestic violence intervention programs. *Addictive Behaviors, 28*, 1603-1610.

Teplin, L. A., McClelland, G. M., & Abram, K. M. (2005). Crime victimization in adults with severe mental illness: Comparison with the National Crime Victimization Survey. *Archives of General Psychiatry, 62,* 911-921.

Tjaden, P., & Thoennes N. (2000). Prevalence and consequences of male-to-female and female-to-male intimate partner violence as measured by the National Violence Against Women Survey. *Violence Against Women, 6,* 142-161.

Tsai, S.-J., Hwang, J.-P., Yang, C.-H., & Liu, K.-M. (1997). Delusional jealousy in dementia. *Journal of Clinical Psychiatry, 58,* 492-494.

Webster, C. D., Douglas, K. S., Eaves, D., & Hart, S. D. (1997). *HCR-20: Assessing Risk for Violence* (Version 2). Burnaby, B. C.: Mental Health, Law, and Policy Institute, Simon Fraser University.`

Wilke, D. J., & Vinton, L. (2005). The nature and impact of domestic violence across age cohorts. *Affilia, 20,* 316-328.

Williams, K. R., & Houghton, A. B. (2004). Assessing the risk of domestic violence reoffending: A validation study. *Law and Human Behavior, 28,* 437-455.

Worthen, J. B., & Varnado-Sullivan, P. (2005). Gender bias in attributions of responsibility for abuse. *Journal of Family Violence, 20,* 305-312.

doi:10.1300/J084v19n01_02

From Behind the Shadows:
A Profile of the Sexual Abuse
of Older Men Residing in Nursing Homes

Pamela B. Teaster, PhD
Holly Ramsey-Klawsnik, PhD
Marta S. Mendiondo, PhD
Erin Abner, MPH
Kara Cecil, BS
Mary Tooms, BS

Pamela B. Teaster is Associate Professor, Graduate Center for Gerontology, 303C Wethington Health Sciences Building, 900 South Limestone, University of Kentucky, Lexington, KY 40536-0200 (E-mail: pteaster@uky.edu). Holly Ramsey-Klawsnik is a Sociologist and Licensed Mental Health Clinician in Private Practice, 24 High Street, Canton, MA 02021 (E-mail: ramsey-klawsnik@comcast.net). Marta S. Mendiondo is Assistant Professor, Biostatistics, 800 South Limestone, University of Kentucky, Lexington, KY 40536-0230 (E-mail: marta@uky.edu). Erin Abner is Data Manager, 800 South Limestone, University of Kentucky, Lexington, KY 40536-0230 (E-mail: elabne@uky.edu). Kara Cecil is Graduate Research Assistant, Graduate Center for Gerontology, 303C Wethington Health Sciences Building, 900 South Limestone, University of Kentucky, Lexington, KY 40536-0200 (E-mail: kara.cecil@uky.edu). Mary Tooms is Graduate Research Assistant, Graduate Center for Gerontology, 303C Wethington Health Sciences Building, 900 South Limestone, University of Kentucky, Lexington, KY 40536-0200 (E-mail: mary.tooms@aol.com).

The authors express their appreciation to APS staff in New Hampshire, Oregon, Tennessee, Texas, and Wisconsin, DADs staff in Texas and Elder Abuse/BQA staff in Wisconsin, and study liaisons (Lynne Koontz, Valerie Eames, Nancy Jackson, Marilyn Whalen, Cynthia Guichet, Jane Raymond, Todd Boerger, and Shari Busse) for assisting with data collection. Support for this study was provided by the National Institute on Aging, R01 AG022944.

[Haworth co-indexing entry note]: "From Behind the Shadows: A Profile of the Sexual Abuse of Older Men Residing in Nursing Homes." Teaster, Pamela B. et al. Co-published simultaneously in *Journal of Elder Abuse & Neglect*™ (The Haworth Maltreatment & Trauma Press®, an imprint of The Haworth Press, Inc.) Vol. 19, No. 1/2, 2007, pp. 29-45; and: *Abuse of Older Men* (ed: Jordan I. Kosberg) The Haworth Maltreatment & Trauma Press®, an imprint of The Haworth Press, Inc., 2007, pp. 29-45. Single or multiple copies of this article are available for a fee from The Haworth Document Delivery Service [1-800-HAWORTH, 9:00 a.m. - 5:00 p.m. (EST). E-mail address: docdelivery@haworthpress.com].

Available online at http://jean.haworthpress.com
doi:10.1300/J084v19n01_03

SUMMARY. Previous research on the sexual abuse of older adults has revealed few cases of the sexual abuse of older men. The first national study of the sexual abuse of vulnerable adults in facilities, reported in this article, collected data on alleged, investigated, and substantiated cases of sexual abuse. This study revealed 26 cases reported and screened in for investigation concerning the alleged sexual abuse of older men (aged 50 and older) residing in nursing homes. Cases occurred in five states within a six month time period. Of these cases, six were confirmed upon investigation by Adult Protective Services or other regulatory agencies. Victims tended to be predominately white males with cognitive and physical deficits that limited their ability for self care. The most typical sexual abuse alleged and substantiated was fondling. Residents were more often substantiated as the abuser than other perpetrators. Sexual abuse of older men in nursing homes crosses traditional gender, cultural, and role boundaries for both victims and perpetrators. doi:10.1300/J084v19n01_03 *[Article copies available for a fee from The Haworth Document Delivery Service: 1-800-HAWORTH. E-mail address: <docdelivery@haworthpress.com> Website: <http://www.HaworthPress.com> © 2007 by The Haworth Press, Inc. All rights reserved.]*

KEYWORDS. Sexual abuse, older men, adult protective services, regulatory entities, elder abuse, abuse in nursing homes

INTRODUCTION

This article discusses findings from the first national study of the sexual abuse of vulnerable adults residing in care facilities. Data were collected from Adult Protective Services (APS) and other regulatory entities from five states involving reported, investigated, and substantiated cases of sexual abuse in a variety of care settings, including nursing homes, assisted living facilities, psychiatric hospitals, state schools for people with developmental disabilities, and community-based residential care facilities. Findings are presented on the sexual abuse of older men residing in nursing homes. The National Clearinghouse on Abuse in Later Life (NCALL) defines older victims as those ages 50 and over (NCALL, 2006). Following NCALL's lead, this paper will report on alleged and confirmed male victims of sexual abuse ages 50 and over (hereafter referred to as "older males").

SEXUAL ABUSE OF OLDER PERSONS

Sexual Abuse

Although all types of elder abuse are purportedly underreported, no abuse is thought to be so underreported as the sexual abuse of older adults (Mickish, 1993; Teaster & Roberto, 2004). Sexual abuse is defined as "non-consenting sexual contact of any kind" (National Center on Elder Abuse [NCEA], 1995, p. 1), and includes unwanted touching; sexual assault or battery, such as rape, sodomy, and coerced nudity; sexually explicit photographing; and sexual contact with any person incapable of giving consent. The range of sexually abusive behavior also includes sexual harassment, threatening rape or molestation, forcing a victim to view pornographic materials, exhibitionism, and harmful genital practices (unnecessary, obsessive or painful touching of the genital area which does not occur as part of a medical or nursing care plan) (Ramsey-Klawsnik, 1991, 1996).

Most research on the sexual abuse of older adults has reported primarily female victims (Burgess et al., 2000; Burgess, Ramsey-Klawsnik & Gregorian, under review; Holt, 1993; Ramsey-Klawsnik, 1991, 1993, 1996, 2003; Roberto, Teaster & Nikzad (in press); Roberto & Teaster, 2005; Teaster, Roberto, Duke, & Kim, 2000; Teaster & Roberto, 2003). An extensive search of the research literature revealed very few studies that report cases of the sexual abuse of older men.

Sexual Abuse in Nursing Homes

Hawes (2003) utilized data from the National Ombudsman Reporting System (NORS) and found that in 1998 long-term care ombudsmen reported approximately 20,000 complaints involving abuse, neglect, or exploitation, and in a two year period, more than 1,700 of which involved complaints of alleged sexual abuse. A General Accounting Office (GAO) report (2002) revealed unacceptable levels of physical and sexual abuse in nursing homes and discussed 158 investigations of physical and sexual abuse in long-term care. Payne and Civokic (1996) examined 488 incidents of abuse of residents in nursing homes derived from *Medicaid Fraud Reports*. They found that 43 out of 488 (8.8%) cases involved sexual abuse.

OLDER MALE VICTIMS OF ABUSE

The paucity of attention given to the abuse of older men in both research and practice literature may stem from empirical findings that, in general, men are more often offenders than the victims of abuse (Kosberg, 1998). Mouton and colleagues (2001) provided a concise literature review of elder abuse and neglect and emphasized the presence of males as victims of elder abuse and neglect. The prevalence study by Pillemer and Finkelhor (1998) found that older men were abused at a *per capita* rate nearly double that of older women. Further, Tatara (1993) examined state APS reports of abuse and found that the proportion of elderly male to elderly female victims of abuse exceeded the proportion of elderly men to elderly women in the general population.

From 1996 to 2006, reports of the abuse of adults over the age of 60 have risen by 30% (Teaster, Otto, Dugar, Mendiondo, Abner, & Cecil, 2006). Reflected in that rise are the types of substantiated abuse, often multiple forms, to which victims are subjected, including physical abuse (7,691 reports or 10.7%), emotional/psychological/verbal abuse (10,656 or 14.8%), self-neglect (26,752 reports or 37.2%), financial exploitation (10,569 or 14.7%), caregiver neglect/abandonment (14,680 or 20.4%), and sexual abuse (742 or 1.0%) (Teaster et al.). The study by Teaster et al. found that 34.3% of all victims were male, and the vast majority (89.3%) of these substantiated abuses occurred in domestic settings. However, the study relied upon data provided by APS systems nationwide. In many states, APS does not have the responsibility or the authority to investigate alleged abuse in facilities, hence substantiated abuses that occurred in nursing homes in many states are not reflected in these national findings.

FINDINGS ON THE SEXUAL ABUSE OF OLDER MEN

Holt (1993) reported on 90 elders in Great Britain who were believed to have been sexually abused, including 13 males. About half of the men had dementia, one-third was stroke victims and one-third was described as frail. The majority of alleged male victims functioned at "poor" or "very poor" levels. In two-thirds of these cases, it was believed by reporting individuals that the victims had been raped. A report of twenty sexually abused nursing home residents (Burgess, Dowdell, & Prentky, 2000) found the majority of victims to be female, with only two identified male victims.

An 18-month examination of cases handled by three social service departments in the north of England identified 186 cases of abuse (Pritchard, 2001). Of these, 39 of the victims were men, 29 of whom were 60 years of age and older. Pritchard conducted in-depth interviews with two of the older men who had experienced sexual abuse. One of the men (age 76) had been sexually abused by his wife. For the second male victim (age 79), a "friend" who cared for, but who did not live with, the victim and his wife physically abused the male victim and also forced sexual activity with "the friend" as well as prostitutes. Both cases highlight the hidden and long-term vulnerability of older men abused by persons they once trusted and upon whom they were reliant for care.

A qualitative analysis of elder sexual abuse that occurred within families (Ramsey-Klawsnik, 2003) found that older husbands are seldom sexually abused by their wives, although cases are occasionally reported, investigated, and substantiated. Older male victims of sexually abusive spouses displayed psycho-social consequences similar to the long-term victimization of females, including low self-esteem and hopelessness. Also, like female victims, males were reported to experience multiple barriers to leaving a long-term violent marriage (such as emotional, social, and financial attachment to the abuser and the perceived duty to remain to care for the spouse).

Burgess, Ramsey-Klawsnik, and Gregorian (under review) report 284 cases of alleged and confirmed sexual abuse of elders that came to official attention through reports to either law enforcement or APS. About one-quarter of the alleged assaults occurred in facilities. The overwhelming majority of suspected victims were female, only 6.5% were male. This study reported fairly typical findings regarding alleged perpetrators, in that the vast majority (90.9%) was male.

Roberto, Teaster, and Nikzad (in press) explored the sexual abuse of vulnerable younger and older men, including the nature of the sexual abuse, characteristics of victims and perpetrators, and case outcomes. Of the 134 cases submitted to researchers, only 17 concerned the sexual abuse of men. Three men lived in the community with at least one family member (e.g., mother, sibling), and four lived in facilities. As a group, the men were limited in personal care abilities due to orientation and ambulation deficits and an inability to manage their own financial affairs. The abuse most frequently experienced was kissing, fondling, and unwelcome interest in their body. In over half the cases, the men experienced multiple forms of sexual abuse. Younger men were victims of a wider range of sexual abuse acts than their middle age and older counterparts. In two instances, the sexual abuse was reported by residents of the facilities in which the men lived. Outcomes for the residents consisted largely of relocation and physical or psychological treatment. Two of the men were judged to remain at risk after APS intervention.

SUMMARY OF ELDER SEXUAL ABUSE LITERATURE

Ramsey-Klawsnik, Teaster, Mendiondo, Abner, Cecil, and Tooms (in press) provide a detailed review of the elder sexual abuse literature. They conclude that available research indicates that this is a problem involving primarily female victims and male perpetrators with few identified male victims and female perpetrators. Victims tend to be highly impaired due to advanced age and physical and cognitive limitations. Perpetrators include family members, paid care providers, and fellow residents in facilities.

Studies of the sexual abuse of adults with disabilities (Brown, Stein, & Turk, 1995; Furey, 1994) have found a higher rate of male victimization than that discovered within the elder abuse field. This raises the possibility that the rate of sexual abuse of men within nursing homes is higher than reported, given that many people living in nursing homes experience significant disabilities. Like their female counterparts, older men who are sexually abused may regard that their ability to exist in an abusive relationship, or to escape it, is severely limited due to the need for assistance with personal care, lack of housing alternatives, or even an inability to recognize abuse at all.

ANALYSIS OF DATA ON SEXUALLY ABUSED OLDER MEN

The purpose of this article is to report on an analysis of APS and other regulatory body investigated and substantiated reports of the sexual abuse of older men in nursing homes in order to understand characteristics of the abuse. The analysis of data sought to answer the following questions: What is the nature of the sexual abuse of older men residing in nursing homes? Who are the older institutionalized male sexual abuse victims and their perpetrators? How are cases investigated, and how are cases substantiated? What are the outcomes of the cases of the sexual abuse of older men in nursing homes?

Methods

Data were collected prospectively concerning suspected and substantiated cases of the sexual abuse of vulnerable adults from May 1, 2005 until October 31, 2005 from contemporaneous reports in the states of New Hampshire, Oregon, Tennessee, Texas, and Wisconsin. For the five states, there were a total of 1961 certified nursing facilities during the study period (State Health Facts, 2007). The research team developed an extensive data collection instrument, the Sex Abuse Survey (SASU), that drew upon earlier work conducted by Ramsey-Klawsnik (1991) and Teaster and Roberto (2004), as well as input from APS and regulatory professionals who piloted the survey and then completed it. In compliance with protections for confidentiality and to ensure the highest quality of information, investigatory staff completed the SASU using case file information for reference. Staff closest to the investigation was asked to complete the SASU as soon as possible after they had closed the investigation. SASUs were submitted to researchers at the University of Kentucky via e-mail, a Web-site specifically designated for data collection purposes, and fax. SASUs also were tracked by liaisons in each state. Fifteen percent of completed SASUs then were checked against the case file by state liaisons in order to ensure accuracy of information provided. State-level administration was highly supportive of the study, but data were submitted by staff on a purely voluntary basis. Data gathered included personal characteristics of the alleged victims and their ability to care for themselves and to communicate; a description of the sexual abuse; witness(es) to the abuse; time spent on, and the nature of, the investigations; the alleged offenders; the resolution of the case; and victim outcomes.

Results

Study findings provide a rich understanding of the complexities involved in the sexual abuse of older men living in nursing homes. Given the small number of cases, and in order to protect confidentiality, information about the men gathered during the six months is presented only in the aggregate form.

Sample. During the data collection period, there were 430 investigations and 91 (21%) substantiations of the sexual abuse of adults 18+ living in facilities, with 177 (41%) investigations and 52 (29%) substantiations of the sexual abuse of men and women 50 years of age and older. Of these alleged older victims, 37 (20%) resided in nursing homes.

There were 26 men older men residing in nursing homes who had allegedly been sexually abused and whose cases were investigated. The sexual
abuse of six of these men was substantiated. The ages of the older men
whose alleged sexual abuse was investigated ranged from 50 to 93 years
of age (mean = 71) (see Table 1). Investigations revealed that 19 (73%)
of the older men were white, and four (15%) were African-Americans.
The sexual abuse substantiation rate for the older men residing in nursing homes was 25%, or roughly half the substantiation rate for all types
of abuse of adults 60 and older, or 46% (Teaster et al., 2006).

Type of Sexual Abuse. Fondling was the most common form of alleged abuse and occurred in 35% of the alleged cases. Inappropriate
sexual behavior related to sexual interest in the victim's body was the
next most common form of alleged abuse (27%) (see Table 2). Fondling
was also the most commonly substantiated abuse.

TABLE 1. Characteristics of Alleged and Substantiated Older Male Victims

	Alleged Victims N = 26	%	Substantiated Victims N = 6	%
Age				
50-59	7	(27%)	1	(17%)
60-69	4	(15%)	2	(33%)
70-79	7	(27%)	0	(0%)
80+	8	(31%)	3	(50%)
Median age	71 years (50-93)		75 years (58-93)	
Race				
White	19	(73%)	5	(83%)
African American	4	(15%)	1	(17%)
Other	1	(4%)	0	(0%)
Unknown	1	(4%)	0	(0%)
Ethnicity				
Not Hispanic/Latino	17	(65%)	5	(83%)
Hispanic/Latino	3	(12%)	0	(0%)
Unknown	3	(12%)	1	(17%)
Missing	3	(12%)	0	(0%)

TABLE 2. Types of Alleged Sexual Abuse of Older Men in Nursing Homes

Abuse	All Victims N = 26	%	Substantiated Victims N = 6	%
Fondling	9	(35%)	4	(67%)
Inappropriate sexual behavior related to sexual interest in victim's body	7	(27%)	1	(17%)
Other	5	(19%)	1	(17%)
Oral genital contact	4	(15%)	0	(0%)
Digital penetration of anus	3	(12%)	0	(0%)
Sexual jokes and comments	2	(8%)	0	(0%)
Anal rape	1	(9%)	1	(17%)
Exposure to embarrass or humiliate	1	(9%)	1	(17%)
Showing victim pornography	1	(9%)	1	(17%)

(Each case may have multiple abuses)

Abilities of the Men. The men tended to be perceived cognitively as fairly well oriented, with over half of investigations involving men oriented to person (85%) and place (54%), and over a third oriented to time (39%). Most of the men (77%) in investigated cases either were not ambulatory or required physical or mechanical assistance. Over half (64%) either needed assistance with their finances or could not manage them. Over half (54%) had no barriers to communication. Abilities and needs of the men in the subset of six substantiated cases were generally similar to those in the larger investigated sample, although all six were reportedly oriented to person all the time (see Table 3).

Nature of Incidents. In 18 investigations (75%) the abuse was reported to be an isolated incident, in two (8%) investigations multiple incidents of abuse were alleged, and in one (4%) investigation there were only signs or symptoms of abuse, but no specific incident was reported. Seven (29%) of the investigated reports were indicated as resident-to-resident sexual contact, considered facility neglect by the investigating agency. Of the six substantiated cases, four (67%) were isolated incidents (including two resident-to-resident cases), one (17%) included signs and symptoms of abuse with no specific incident, and one (17%) case was reported only as resident-to-resident sexual contact. In 11 (38%) of the 24 cases, there was no witness to the abuse. Where the witnesses' relationship to the alleged victim was known, staff witnessed the abuse in seven (29%) cases, and in one instance another nursing home resident was a witness. For substantiated cases, there was no witness in two (33%)

TABLE 3. Abilities of Alleged and Substantiated Older Male Victims of Sexual Abuse

	All Victims N = 26	%	Substantiated Victims N = 6	%
Orientation to Person				
All of the time	22	(85%)	6	(100%)
Some of the time	1	(4%)	0	(0%)
None of the time	1	(4%)	0	(0%)
Missing	2	(8%)	0	(0%)
Orientation to Place				
All of the time	14	(54%)	2	(50%)
Some of the time	4	(15%)	1	(17%)
None of the time	4	(15%)	1	(17%)
Missing	4	(15%)	2	(33%)
Orientation to Time				
All of the time	10	(39%)	2	(33%)
Some of the time	6	(23%)	2	(33%)
None of the time	7	(27%)	1	(17%)
Missing	3	(12%)	1	(17%)
Ambulation				
Without assistance	3	(12%)	1	(17%)
Physical/Mechanical assistance	17	(65%)	4	(67%)
Not ambulatory	4	(15%)	1	(17%)
Missing	2	(8%)	0	(0%)
Management of Finances				
Alone	1	(3%)	1	(17%)
With assistance	2	(8%)	0	(0%)
Unable to manage	15	(58%)	4	(67%)
Unknown	8	(31%)	1	(17%)
Ability to Communicate				
No barriers to communication	14	(54%)	4	(67%)
Verbal, but with difficulty	7	(27%)	0	(0%)
Only non-verbal	1	(4%)	0	(0%)
Unable to communicate	1	(4%)	1	(17%)
Unknown	3	(12%)	1	(17%)

of the cases, and staff witnessed the sexual abuse in four cases (67%). Injuries either did not occur or were not discovered.

The Alleged Perpetrator. The alleged perpetrator was identified in 96% of the investigations and in 100% of substantiated cases. Over half (54%) of the alleged offenders were male, and 83% of the substantiated offenders were male (see Table 4). Females were alleged perpetrators in

TABLE 4. Characteristics of Alleged Perpetrators of Sexual Abuse of Older Men in Nursing Homes

	All Cases N = 24	%	Substantiated Cases N = 6	%
Age				
18-39	9	(38%)	0	(0%)
40-59	7	(29%)	2	(33%)
60-79	4	(17%)	3	(50%)
80+	0	(0%)	0	(0%)
Missing	4	(17%)	1	(17%)
Mean age	36 years (20-60)		61 years (56-68)	
Gender				
Male	13	(54%)	5	(83%)
Female	10	(42%)	1	(17%)
Missing	1	(4%)	0	(0%)
Race				
White	11	(46%)	4	(67%)
African American	7	(29%)	0	(0%)
Unknown	4	(17%)	1	(17%)
Other	2	(8%)	1	(17%)
Ethnicity				
Not Hispanic or Latino	13	(54%)	4	(67%)
Unknown	8	(33%)	1	(17%)
Hispanic or Latino	3	(13%)	1	(17%)
Relationship to victim				
Facility staff	16	(75%)	0	(0%)
Resident/client in facility	6	(25%)	4	(67%)
Family member	1	(4%)	1	(17%)
Unknown	1	(4%)	1	(17%)

10 investigated cases and the substantiated abuser in one case. In investigations, 25% of alleged perpetrators were other residents of the facility. Of these, one perpetrator allegedly victimized three residents. In substantiated cases, residents constituted 67% of perpetrators. Although a staff member was identified as the perpetrator in 75% of investigated reports, none were confirmed as perpetrators.

Resolution of the Case. It was not uncommon for several agencies to be involved with cases of sexual abuse. APS or a regulatory entity solely investigated 65% cases and jointly investigated 35% of the cases with other entities (e.g., law enforcement, the ombudsman, and other regulatory entities). Time spent in investigation ranged from 2 to 18 hours, with a mean of 9 hours. For substantiated reports, investigations ranged from 4.5 to 8 hours, with a mean of 6.2 hours.

Case Outcomes. Interventions or services were provided for victims of both investigated and substantiated cases (see Table 5). For the 26 men, five received care plan changes, four received a nursing evaluation, two were moved within the facility, and nine received no intervention. Of the six substantiated victims, two had their care plans changed, one received a nursing care evaluation, one was moved within the facility, and one received sexual abuse prevention intervention. Half of the men confirmed were deemed to be at continued risk of further sexual abuse by the

TABLE 5. Interventions for Alleged and Substantiated Older Male Victims of Sexual Abuse in Nursing Homes

Intervention	All Victims N = 26	%	Substantiated Victims N = 6	%
None	9	(35%)	0	(0%)
Care plan changed	5	(19%)	2	(33%)
Nursing care evaluation	4	(15%)	1	(17%)
Moved victim within facility	2	(8%)	1	(17%)
Case management counseling	1	(4%)	0	(0%)
Alternative housing	1	(4%)	0	(0%)
Hospitalization	1	(4%)	0	(0%)
Supervision increased	1	(4%)	0	(0%)
Mental health counseling	1	(4%)	0	(0%)
Sexual abuse prevention	1	(4%)	1	(17%)

(Victims can receive multiple interventions)

perpetrator. Half of the perpetrators were relocated. In no substantiated cases was there an arrest of the perpetrator.

DISCUSSION AND CONCLUSION

The 24 investigated and six substantiated cases of sexual abuse of older men residing in nursing homes revealed that, as a group, most of the alleged and confirmed victims were white men who had limitations in personal care abilities due to orientation and/or ambulation deficits, and an inability to manage their own financial affairs. Overall, the characteristics of the men were similar to those victims in earlier studies (e.g., Burgess, Dowdell, & Prentky, 2000; Ramsey-Klawsnik, 1991, 2003; Roberto & Teaster, 2005; Teaster & Roberto, 2003); that is, all were vulnerable to abuse due to mental and/or physical deficits. That most of the men in earlier studies were white suggests that there may be gender as well as cultural differences to address when working cases of this nature.

The type of sexual abuse most frequently substantiated was fondling, but other forms were also substantiated, including inappropriate behavior related to sexual interest in the victim's body, exposure of private body parts to harass or humiliate, and showing the victim pornography. One case of anal rape was substantiated. In eight investigations, and three substantiations, multiple forms of sexual abuse were alleged. Again, these phenomena are consistent with findings in earlier studies (Roberto, Teaster & Nikzad, in press; Teaster & Roberto, 2004). Because many of the residents were oriented to person and time, it seems critical that residents and their families understand their rights, one of which is to live in an environment free from abuse and neglect (Stahlman & Kisor, 2000).

Little literature exists concerning female sexual offenders. Of significant interest, ten of the 23 alleged sexual perpetrators were female, and one woman was confirmed as a perpetrator. Sixteen of the 23 alleged perpetrators were staff members of the facilities who provided care to the alleged victims; however, none of them were confirmed as perpetrators. Four of the six alleged perpetrators, who were fellow residents, were confirmed as abusers. These findings raise an important question: Is it easier, for whatever reason, for investigators to confirm a facility resident as a sexual offender rather than to substantiate a facility staff member as a perpetrator?

In 18 of 24 investigations, the abuse was regarded as an isolated incident, and in two cases the abuse was alleged to be ongoing over a period of time. Staff reported witnessing sexual abuse in seven situations, and a nursing home resident was a witness in one case. It is somewhat surprising that only six cases were substantiated (including two that involved no witnesses) given that eight cases involved witnessed sexual abuse.

APS alone investigated well over half of all the cases and with other entities in nine of the cases. Due to the complex nature of sexual abuse, which is often accompanied by other forms of abuse and which frequently constitutes criminal activity, it is recommended that APS work in concert with other appropriate entities during the investigatory process. Collaboration with medical and legal professionals may increase successful prosecutions when a sexual crime has been committed. Law enforcement should be involved in appropriate cases involving the sexual abuse of a resident by a fellow resident, as he or she, if competent, may well be guilty of a crime.

Services for the men consisted largely of care plan changes and relocation within the nursing homes. It may be that other interventions were necessary, but–if provided–occurred after the completion of this study. It is suspected that this is the case. At the time data were collected, three of the substantiated sexual abuse victims were judged to be at risk for further victimization, and the research team was unable to gather information on the reasons these men remained at risk. If the risk is of their choosing, and if the men are competent to make decisions, then such risk, while it may be viewed to be unfortunate, preserves the autonomy of the men. However, if their safety is compromised due to problems in the facility, or problems on a wider and systemic scale, then protective mechanisms have failed them. Interventions to swiftly remove them from "at risk" situations are then critical. While the preservation of individual autonomy needs to be affirmed, there may be instances when preservation of autonomy obfuscates a duty to protect a vulnerable individual from harm. Such situations represent profoundly complex ethical, legal, clinical, and public policy issues.

As with earlier studies on this topic, we recognize four limitations to this study. First, data on sexual abuse cases were provided by APS or regulatory staff, and there might have been errors made in completing data collection tools. This was possible, even though care was taken in the study to train staff in each state on data collection and to review data provided for accuracy. Second, based on estimates from the *National Elder Abuse Incidence Study*, elder abuse cases reported to APS represent only about 16% of the actual number of incidents (Dunlop, Rothman, Condon, Hebert, & Martinez, 2000). Suggested earlier, due to the nature of this type of abuse, unreported incidences of sexual abuse may be far higher. Hence, sexual abuse of vulnerable adults may well be greater in scope than that presented by our data. Moreover, because the sexual abuse of women is more readily understood than the sexual abuse of men, reports concerning men may occur far less frequently than other forms of abuse in which men are involved and for which easier remedies exist. Third, though information was requested on all investigated reports of sexual abuse within a specified timeframe, information was submitted at the discretion of staff.

Finally, APS and other regulatory agencies with the authority to investigate alleged sexual abuse must find sufficient evidence in order to substantiate a reported case. Investigatory agencies involved in the cases described in this paper substantiated six out of 24 alleged cases of the sexual abuse of older men in nursing homes. The 18 alleged but unsubstantiated may include actual cases of sexual abuse in which insufficient evidence emerged during the investigation to justify a positive finding. There are many reasons why evidence of actual abuse may become lost or contaminated, including witnesses and victims fearful of retaliation who do not disclose or may recant statements, delayed or missing physical examinations of alleged victims, and sexual abuse perpetrators who are motivated to lie and hide evidence of their crimes. Thus, our study does not report the actual number of incidences of sexual abuse in nursing homes during the study time period. Rather, it contains only those cases actually reported to state authorities and investigated and those that could be substantiated. It does not include unreported cases.

Despite limitations, this study represents the first prospective and systematic study of the sexual abuse of vulnerable adults in facilities in the country. Its aggregate numbers include more male victims than any other published study on the topic to date. For the future, researchers must become aware of, and understand, the sexual abuse of vulnerable adults within institutional and community settings. Research should address whether allegations, investigations, and substantiations of the sexual abuse of men are substantively different from those of women, from those of younger versus older victims, and of those in various care settings. Also for future consideration, there are a number of questions: What is the appropriate response of facilities and agencies when addressing allegations of sexual abuse of older men by residents versus members of the staff? Who are the most appropriate investigators of such cases? What are long-term consequences for and outcomes of interventions for victims? What are appropriate interventions for perpetrators?

In conclusion, the findings reveal, first and foremost, that the sexual abuse of older men in nursing homes does occur. Sexual abuse crosses traditional gender, cultural, and role boundaries for victims and perpetrators and underscores a need for specialized training and intervention efforts by APS, law enforcement, and medical and mental health care providers involved in diverse care settings.

REFERENCES

Brown, H., Stein, J., & Turk, S. (1995). The sexual abuse of adults with learning disabilities: Report of a second two-year incidence survey. *Mental Handicap Research, 8*, 3-24.

Burgess, A. W., Brown, K., Bell, K., Ledray, L. E., & Poarch, J. C. (2005). Sexual abuse of older adults: Assessing for signs of a serious crime–and reporting it. *American Journal of Nursing, 105*(10), 66-71.

Burgess, A. W., Dowdel, E. B., & Prentky, R. A. (2000). Sexual abuse of nursing home residents. *Journal of Psychosocial Nursing and Mental Health Services, 36*(6), 10-18.

Dunlop, B. D., Rothman, M. B., Condon, K. M., Hebert, K. S., & Martinez, I. L. (2000). Elder abuse: Risk factors and use of case data to improve policy and practice. *Journal of Elder Abuse & Neglect, 12*(3/4), 95-122.

Furey, E. M. (1994). Sexual abuse of adults with mental retardation: Who and where. *Mental Retardation, 32*, 173-180.

General Accounting Office (2002). *Nursing homes: More can be done to protect residents from abuse.* Washington, DC: US General Accounting Office.

Hawes, C. (2003). Elder abuse in residential long-term care settings: What is known and what information is needed? In R. J. Bonnie & R. B. Wallace (Eds.), *Elder mistreatment: Abuse, neglect and exploitation in aging America* (pp. 446-500). Washington, DC: The National Academies Press.

Holt, M. G. (1993). Elder sexual abuse in Britain: Preliminary findings. *Journal of Elder Abuse & Neglect, 5*(2), 63-71.

Kosberg, J. I. (1998). The abuse of elderly men. *Journal of Elder Abuse & Neglect, 9*(3), 69-88.

Mickish, J. (1993). Abuse and neglect: The adult and elder. In B. Byers & J. Hendricks (Eds.), *Adult protective service: Reach and practice* (pp. 33-60). Springfield, IL: Charles C. Thomas.

Mouton, C. P., Talamantes, M., Parker, R. W., Espino, D. V., & Miles, T. P. (2001). Abuse and neglect in older men. *Clinical Gerontologist, 24*(3-4), 15-26.

National Center on Elder Abuse. (1995). Elder abuse in a domestic settings. *Elder Abuse Information Series #3.* Retrieved March 14, 2003, from http://www.elderabusecenter. org/basic/fact3.pdf

National Clearinghouse on Abuse in Later Life (2006). Definitions. Retrieved December 9, 2006, from http://www.ncall.us

Payne, B., & Civokic, R. (1996). An empirical examination of the characteristics, consequences, and causes of elder abuse in nursing homes. *Journal of Elder Abuse & Neglect, 7*(4), 61-74.

Pillemer, K. A., & Finkelhor, D. (1988). The prevalence of elder abuse: A random sample survey. *The Gerontologist, 28*, 51-57.

Pritchard, J. (2001). *Male victims of elder abuse: Their experiences and needs.* London: Jessica Kingsley Publishers.

Ramsey-Klawsnik, H. (1991). Elder sexual abuse: Preliminary findings. *Journal of Elder Abuse & Neglect, 3*(3), 73-90.

Ramsey-Klawsnik, H. (1993). Interviewing elders for suspected sexual abuse: Guidelines and techniques. *Journal of Elder Abuse & Neglect, 5*(1), 5-18.

Ramsey-Klawsnik, H. (1996). Assessing physical and sexual abuse in health care settings. In L. Baumhover & S.C. Beal (Eds.), *Abuse, neglect, and exploitation of older persons: Strategies for assessment and intervention* (pp. 67-87). Baltimore, MD: Health Professions Press.

Ramsey-Klawsnik, H. (2003). Elder sexual abuse within the family. *Journal of Elder Abuse & Neglect, 15*(1), 43-58.

Roberto, K. A., & Teaster, P. B. (2005). Sexual abuse of vulnerable young and old women: A comparative analysis of circumstances and outcomes. *Violence Against Women, 11*, 473-504.

Roberto, K. A., Teaster, P. B., & Nikzad, K. (under review). Sexual abuse of vulnerable adult men. *Interpersonal Violence.*

Stahlman, S., & Kisor, A. (2000). Nursing homes. In R. Schneider, N. Kropf, & A. Kisor (Eds.), *Gerontological social work: Knowledge, service settings, and special populations* (2nd ed.) (pp. 225-254). Belmont, CA: Brooks/Cole.

State Health Facts. (2007). Health facts. Retrieved January 10, 2007, from http://www.statehealthfacts.org/cgi-bin/healthfacts

Tatara, T. (1993). Understanding the nature and scope of domestic elder abuse with the use of state aggregate data: Summaries of the key findings of a national survey of state APS and aging agencies. *Journal of Elder Abuse & Neglect, 5*(4), 35-51.

Teaster, P. B., & Roberto, K. A. (2004). The sexual abuse of older adults: APS cases and outcomes. *The Gerontologist, 44*(6), 788-796.

Teaster, P. B., & Roberto, K. A. (2003). Sexual abuse of older women living in nursing homes. *Journal of Gerontological Social Work, 4*, 105-137.

Teaster, P. B., Roberto, K. A., Duke, J. O., & Kim, M. (2000). Sexual abuse of older adults: Preliminary findings of cases in Virginia. *Journal of Elder Abuse & Neglect, 12*(3/4), 17-51.

Teaster, P. B., Otto, J. M., Dugar, T. D., Mendiondo, M. S., Abner, E. L., & Cecil, K. A. (2006). The 2004 survey of state Adult Protective Services: Abuse of adults 60 years of age and older. Report to the National Center on Elder Abuse, Administration on Aging, Washington, D.C.

doi:10.1300/J084v19n01_03

Detection and Prevalence
of Abuse of Older Males:
Perspectives from Family Practice

Mark J. Yaffe, MD, MClSc
Deborah Weiss, MSc
Christina Wolfson, PhD
Maxine Lithwick, MSW

Mark J. Yaffe is associated with McGill University, the Department of Family Medicine and St. Mary's Hospital Centre, 3830 Lacombe Avenue, Montreal, Quebec, Canada H3T 1M5 (E-mail: mark.yaffe@mcgill.ca). Deborah Weiss is associated with McGill University, the Departments of Epidemiology, Biostatistics and Occupational Health, 1025 Pine Avenue West, Room P2.028, Montreal, Quebec, Canada, H3A 1A1 (E-mail: deborah.weiss@mail.mcgill.ca). Christina Wolfson is associated with McGill University, the Departments of Epidemiology, Biostatistics and Occupational Health, and Medicine, 1025 Pine Avenue West, Room P2.028, Montreal, Quebec, Canada, H3A 1A1 (E-mail: christina.wolfson@mcgill.ca). Maxine Lithwick is associated with McGill University, Department of Social Work, and Centre de Service Santé et Sociaux Cavendish, CLSC Rene Cassin, 5800 Cavendish Boulevard, Montreal, Quebec, Canada H4W 2T5 (E-mail: maxine.lithwick.cvd@ssss.gouv.qc.ca).

Corresponding author for contact information: Dr. Mark J. Yaffe, Department of Family Medicine, St. Mary's Hospital Centre, 3830 Lacombe Avenue, Montreal, Quebec, Canada, H3T 1M5 (E-mail: mark.yaffe@mcgill.ca).

This study was funded by a grant (MOP-57847) from the Canadian Institutes of Health Research. Appreciation is expressed to Ms. Silvia Straka and Dr. Elizabeth Podnieks for help in the preparation of the grant submission and on theoretical constructs for elder abuse. The cooperation and participation of physicians and staff of St. Mary's Hospital Centre, Sir Mortimer B. Davis Jewish General Hospital and the CLSC Rene Cassin were essential to the operationalization of this project.

[Haworth co-indexing entry note]: "Detection and Prevalence of Abuse of Older Males: Perspectives from Family Practice." Yaffe, Mark J. et al. Co-published simultaneously in *Journal of Elder Abuse & Neglect™* (The Haworth Maltreatment & Trauma Press®, an imprint of The Haworth Press, Inc.) Vol. 19, No. 1/2, 2007, pp. 47-60; and: *Abuse of Older Men* (ed: Jordan I. Kosberg) The Haworth Maltreatment & Trauma Press®, an imprint of The Haworth Press, Inc., 2007, pp. 47-60. Single or multiple copies of this article are available for a fee from The Haworth Document Delivery Service [1-800-HAWORTH, 9:00 a.m. - 5:00 p.m. (EST). E-mail address: docdelivery@haworthpress.com].

SUMMARY. Family doctors' frequent contact with seniors put them in reasonable positions to detect elder abuse and initiate referral to adult protective services. Since doctor reporting is low, however, this paper explores whether the gender of patient and/or doctor impacts on identification of elder mistreatment, or creates differential detection of one gender over the other. Use of the validated Elder Abuse Suspicion Index (EASI), and a structured social work evaluation, is described to provide some gender-based data from Canadian family practice. Specifically, while the prevalence of elder abuse is estimated to range from 12.0% to 13.3%, the specific prevalence was found for females to be 13.6% to 15.2% and for males 9.1% to 9.7%. doi:10.1300/J084v19n01_04 *[Article copies available for a fee from The Haworth Document Delivery Service: 1-800-HAWORTH. E-mail address: <docdelivery@haworthpress.com> Website: <http://www.HaworthPress.com> © 2007 by The Haworth Press, Inc. All rights reserved.]*

KEYWORDS. Elder abuse, older men, family medicine, abuse prevalence

INTRODUCTION

It has been suggested that the needs of heterosexual males have been neglected by the social work profession (Kosberg, 2002) and particular concerns have been voiced about the adequacy of professional response to older men (Kosberg, 2005). This extends to elder abuse where challenges have been made to the common view that women are the clearly predominant victims of such mistreatment (Mouton, Talamantes, Parker, Espino, & Miles, 2001). The questioning of traditional beliefs seems reasonable given that some statistics on elder mistreatment have been derived from studies that differ in definitions of elder abuse used, types of populations surveyed, methodologies used, and mechanisms to identify and report abuse.

The observation that older men are more likely than women to be victims of neglect (especially abandonment) suggests that more rigor is required when considering gender prevalence for elder abuse (Mouton et al., 2001). For example, Pritchard's (2001) British study of victims of elder mistreatment followed by social services identified likely professional bias towards men in that male compared to female victims of elder abuse received fewer holistic assessments (medical, psychological, social). The men reported social workers and police did not take their concerns seriously and provided only limited advice about housing, finances, and legal issues. Further, for the abused men there was less contact with the aforementioned professionals (despite–contrary to male stereotyping–a willingness to talk about the abuse experience) and less likelihood of follow-up, usual abuse protocols were often not utilized, and there were fewer opportunities for victims to make informed choices. Within this context, extrapolating from results in the evolving domestic violence literature, one finds additional reason to believe that males, as victims of elder abuse, may be under-identified, under-reported, and/or receive inadequate care.

There is therefore a need to improve the identification of elder abuse for men. This paper will examine the general role that physicians can assume in such detection and will more specifically explore the role that gender-related factors for both doctor and patient might play in mistreatment detection. Finally, with a view to increasing the understanding of males as victims of elder abuse, the paper will present gender specific prevalence data on such abuse, as collected in a Canadian family practice setting.

PHYSICIAN ROLE IN ELDER ABUSE DETECTION

Identification of elder abuse might improve if those most in contact with seniors are better able to recognize it. Doctors (in particular, family physicians) have great potential for elder abuse detection (Tomlin, 1988) and awareness promotion (Bloom, Ansell, & Bloom, 1989), since they are in contact with their elderly patients, on average, five times per year (Harrell et al., 2002). These professionals, however, tend to view such detection with reservation, and their reporting rate may be as low as 2% (O'Brien, 1986). Reasons for this include absence of clear-cut definitions of elder abuse (Kozak, Elmslie, & Verdon, 1995), validated identification tools, and sufficient time (Jones, Veensta, Seamon, & Krohmer, 1997). Such factors might explain why a mail survey of 2000 American family doctors and internists found 72% of respondents reported receiving no training on elder abuse, 63% had never or almost never asked about it, more than half had never identified a case, and their elicited guesses on the prevalence for elder abuse were less than 25% of published findings (Kennedy, 2005). Furthermore, once detected, most physicians do not know what to do with identified abuses (Lachs & Pillemer, 2004).

GENDER AS A DETERMINANT IN PRIMARY CARE

As the results of the British study described above suggest possible variance in social workers' approach to elder abuse, one wonders whether gender may play a role as well in physician detection and reporting of such mistreatment. While published literature on this is lacking, the roles that patient gender and doctor gender play, either separately or in combination, in routine diagnostic and treatment processes and in health care communication, may shed some light on this. We therefore conducted a systematic, computerized English language literature review using Medline (January 1, 1966 to July 1, 2006) and PsychInfo (January 1, 1985 to July 1, 2006). Search terms included physician-patient relations, sex distribution, male, female, male and female differences, gender identity, patient gender, physician practice patterns, and therapeutic processes. While some of the earlier studies (that is, published prior to 1993) have a number of methodological limitations (Gabbard-Alley, 1995), interesting themes emerge from these and more recent works.

Patient Gender Differences

Gender differences in patients' help-seeking behaviors may influence how doctors view and approach them. For example, studies from diverse parts of the world have shown that women consult doctors more often than men, even when adjustments are made for maternity visits (McWhinney, 1989). Such a pattern may have the effect of biasing physicians to perceive elder abuse as predominantly a woman's problem. Further, within American, Canadian, and British family practice, the top reasons for males seeking health care is comparable, as it is for females, but those causes for men and women differ (McWhinney). Since doctors investigate and diagnose partially on the basis of probabilities, such a differential presentation again may influence how doctors interpret the presentation of signs and symptoms associated either with illness or with elder abuse.

Given the discomfort and/or reluctance that victims of elder abuse often feel in discussing their situations, it is worthwhile to consider patient-related gender communication and behavioral factors that may impact on the treating physician. For example, when, how, or if patients raise developmental lifespan changes for discussion with doctors may be gender-related (Reiser & Rosen, 1984). As well, verbal and non-verbal communication may vary, as words may have different meanings for each gender and each may have different ways of trying to say the same thing (e.g., in discussion of feelings or expressions of pain). Doctors' observations and their methods of de-coding patients' words and cues, feelings, judgments, and counter-transferences may also vary by patient gender (Reiser & Rosen, 1984; McWhinney, 1989). Further, doctors also appear to be influenced by the different sick roles that male and female patients play (e.g., males stereotypically with illness, while initially stoic, may take on dependency roles) (McWhinney).

Patient gender-specific expectations of the doctor-patient dyadic encounter also may affect how the patient communicates with a physician and vice versa. For example, in a large US national survey exploring satisfaction with ambulatory family practice care, women were more likely to be satisfied with physician–related issues, while men were more likely to be satisfied with issues related to process (Wolosin, 2005). There are complementary findings in Norwegian general practice, where for men presenting somatic complaints that were likely related to a psychosocial problem, the overt reason for the encounter was the only factor that influenced disclosure (Gulgrandsen, Fugelli, & Hjortdahl, 1998). Hence, alone or in combination, the aforementioned gender-related factors challenge doctors in their diagnostic process.

Patient Gender and Medical Care Delivery

To appreciate the potential for patient gender to affect physician identification and response to elder abuse, it is instructive to examine other aspects of health care where such bias has been clearly noted. Coronary artery disease (CAD) has received particular attention. For example, amongst those in Israel with CAD, men have been shown to receive more aggressive secondary prevention (e.g., medications to lower serum fats and to reduce risk of new blood vessel obstruction) than women (Abuful, Gidron, & Henkin, 2005). In a study of Canadian patients referred to cardiologists for evaluation of possible new CAD, women overall underwent less non-invasive and invasive testing than did the men (Jaglal, Slaughter, Baigrie, Morgan, & Naylor, 1995). In another Canadian study that followed male and female survivors of heart attacks, care for women was found to decrease with increasing age. However, despite these differences in care, long term survival for women was higher, suggesting possible differences in biological determinants between men and women, and hence possibly validating differences in approach to gender (Alter, Naylor, Austin, & Tu, 2002). In the southeastern United States, women with high blood pressure (a CAD risk factor) have been observed to have their cholesterol (another risk factor) tested less often than men and, when found to be abnormal, to be treated less frequently (Hendrix, Riehle, & Egan, 2005). Also within the American health care setting, when patients of both sexes present with chest pain, physicians' average estimates of the probability of CAD were observed to be higher in men, as was the rate of invasive investigation (Schulman et al., 1999). In England, in a study that followed people with active chest pain due to problems in heart circulation, women were less likely than men to receive tests that might lead to improvement in blood flow (Raine, Crayford, Chan, & Chambers, 1999). An American study reporting similar findings interpreted such differences as possibly being due to men being over-treated, rather than women being inadequately treated (Morabia, Fabre, & Dunand, 1992).

Such apparent differential care based on patient gender also has been described under different circumstances and for other conditions. For example, physicians appear to infantilize older patients more often than younger patients, and this occurs more often for female patients than for males (O'Donnell, 2003). When dealing with a non age-related preventative intervention such as smoking cessation, findings from a cross-sectional mail self-administered survey of Australian general practitioners suggested that doctors are more likely to initiate an opportunistic discussion about smoking cessation with male patients than with female ones (Young & Ward, 1998). In the management of neck pain, Swedish women received more somatic diagnoses, drugs, and consultations with physiotherapists and orthopedists than men, while the latter received more blood tests (Hamberg, Risberg, Johansson, & Westman, 2002).

In mental health care, audiotape reviews of primary care encounters suggest that patients who rate their emotional health poorly tend more often to initiate discussion of depression and, within that subgroup, women do it more often than men (Sleuth & Rubin, 2002). Women with high scores on the Beck Depression Inventory have been found to be statistically significantly more likely to have their depression diagnosed by their primary care doctors than men (Bertakis et al., 2001). When such gender analysis is extended to the actual management of major depression in an out-patient setting, no particular combination of gender of patient and therapist has been reported to affect the process and outcome of therapy (Zlotnick, Elkin, & Shea, 1998).

Physician Gender as a Determinant of Care

Family physicians demonstrate selective awareness of the psychosocial problems affecting their patients (Yaffe & Stewart, 1985; Gulbrandsen,

Hjortdahl, & Fugelli, 1999), and gender of the doctor may be one of the factors that influence this selectivity (Gulbrandsen et al., 1999). Approaches to health care delivery also may be gender dependent. For example, in the realm of occupational health, in the 6-28 week post injury period critical for interventions to prevent long-term disability, certification for sickness for men by male general practitioners in the UK had a statistically significantly higher prevalence than for women by female doctors (Shiels & Gabby, 2006). In carrying out sexual histories, both male and female physicians responding to a self-administered mail survey were significantly more likely to report discomfort taking such history from the same sex patient than with an opposite sex patient (Burd, Nevadunsky, & Bachmann, 2006).

In care provided by 138 US family doctors to 3,256 patients, while no differences were observed in gender neutral screening by male or female doctors, female physicians were statistically significantly more current with health behavior counseling and immunizations for both patient genders (Flocke & Gilchrist, 2005). In an American cross-sectional study that recruited subjects using random digit dialing and relied on patient self-report, both male and female respondents indicated receiving more general screening and counseling services from female physicians than from male physicians. In this same study, female patients reported receiving more gender specific screening from the women doctors, but this benefit did not extend to men seeing women doctors (Henderson & Weisman, 2001).

In routine outpatient medical visits, female doctors conducted longer visits, made more positive and reflective comments, and smiled and nodded more (Hall, Irish, Roter, Ehrlich, & Miller, 1994a). A cross-sectional survey of Australian final-year medical students found both genders more attuned to the concerns of their own gender (Zaharias, Piterman, & Liddell, 2004). Finally, it has been observed that older patients are more likely to be treated in a bio-psycho-social perspective when treated by a physician of the same gender (O'Donnell, 2003). In summary, this literature, though sometimes contradictory, suggests that it may be inappropriate to view the ability or inability of physicians to detect and respond to elder abuse as homogeneous given the findings that physician gender may influence other aspects of health care.

Patients' Attitudes as Related to Physicians' Gender

What of physicians' gender on patients' views of the care that they receive? Our literature review did not identify studies from the primary health care setting that specifically addressed older male responses to male versus female physicians. Anecdotally, the feminization of the medical profession has appeared to be a source of discomfort for some men not accustomed to receiving care and physical examination by women. As well, a study of both hospital outpatient and community encounters of doctor-adult patient (not age stratified) pairs in the US and Canada reported overall satisfaction lowest in the female physician-male patient dyads (Hall, Irish, Roter, Ehrlich, & Miller, 1994b). One might thus hypothesize some reluctance on the part of older men to divulge intimate issues such as elder abuse to female doctors (Gulbrandsen, Hjortdahl, & Fugelli, 1999).

A TOOL TO ASSIST PHYSICIAN DETECTION OF ELDER ABUSE

There are numerous factors that may contribute to the low involvement of physicians in detecting elder abuse, including the possibility that gender bias exists in physician–patient encounters. Accordingly, an effort in Montreal was initiated to improve physician identification of elder abuse through the development of a short, objective, doctor-friendly instrument that could be used by physicians seeing cognitively intact seniors in an ambulatory office setting. Known as the Elder Abuse Suspicion Index (EASI), this six item questionnaire seeks to improve a doctor's suspicion about the presence of elder abuse (Yaffe, Wolfson, Lithwick, & Weiss, 2006). It consists of one question that addresses dependency (a possible abuse risk factor), and 5 questions that focus on signs or symptoms of an older person's mistreatment: financial abuse, material and emotional deprivation, verbal and psychological abuse, and physical and sexual abuse. In the validation of the EASI, 104 family doctors (working either in two university-affiliated family medicine centers or in one government–run community health clinic), administered the EASI in the course of routine office care to 906 cognitively intact adults aged 65 and over who consented to be part of our study.

Of those 906 seniors it was possible to do secondary analyses on gender issues for 858 of them. Our sample was comparable to the general Canadian seniors' population in relation to mental and physical health. Specifically, mean scores on the Mental and Physical Comportment Scales of the Short Form Health Survey (SF-12) were similar to the Canadian normative data for the longer SF-36 (Hopman et al., 2000). The sample also exhibited the traditional 2:1 female to male ratio of visits commonly reported in family practice. Of the 858 subjects available for analysis, 538 (62.7%) were female and 320 (37.3%) were male.

Elder Abuse Prevalence Data Derived from the EASI

It was found that females were significantly more likely than males to respond positively on the EASI question that assessed dependency (70.3% females compared to 29.7% males, $p < 0.05$). Using the responses on the EASI, it was determined that there was suspicion of elder abuse when there was a positive answer on at least one of the remaining five questions that addressed the abuse domains listed above. Only the frequency of a positive response to the question addressing doctors' observations of overt physical signs, or manifested behaviors often associated with elder abuse, was significantly higher in women than men ($p = 0.01$). Using the EASI questions as defined above, the estimated prevalence of elder abuse was 13.2% (113/858). Statistically significant differences ($p = .02$) were found in specific estimates for females at 15.2% (82/538) and for males at 9.7% (31/320).

Characteristics of Males Suspected of Elder Abuse

No statistically significant findings were obtained when the impact of age, education, living status, and primary language were examined for presence or absence of suspected abuse in males versus females. As well, there was no difference found on the Physical Comportment Scale of the SF-12 between males suspected of being abused on the EASI and those not so identified, nor for women suspected of being abused when compared to women not so identified. In contrast, on the SF-12 Mental Comportment Scale both genders showed statistically significant lower scores for the same gender suspected abused vs. non-abused, but the magnitude of the difference was greater for men. For males, non-abused had a mean score of 54.6, suspected abused had a mean score of 48.4 ($p < 0.001$). For females, non-abused had a mean score of 54.4, suspected abused had a mean score of 51.0 ($p = 0.005$). In addition to the objective health rating derived from the SF-12, patients provided a subjective assessment of their health on a six point rating scale (from 1 being "very poor" to 6 being "excellent"). No differences by gender were seen when scores for those suspected of being abused were compared to scores for those non-abused, while both male and female suspected victims were significantly less inclined ($p = 0.02$ and 0.04, respectively) to view their health in a positive light. These health findings are consistent with the elder abuse risk factor literature that associates poorer mental health of seniors with elder abuse victimization. Additionally they support the observations of others (Pritchard, 2001) that the mental health needs of older men deserve more attention. Since our findings come from a family practice setting, there is a challenge for family physicians to be more attentive to this reality.

Elder Abuse Prevalence Data from Social Worker Assessments

Our study on the development and validation of the EASI permitted us to consider elder abuse and gender impact from another perspective. Following family doctor administration of the EASI to their study patient participants, these individuals later underwent a structured 1.5 to 3 hour elder abuse assessment by social workers specifically trained for the task. That encounter used a well-utilized questionnaire developed by the Elder Abuse Centre of the CLSC René Cassin (a health and social service agency) in Montreal, a referral centre for elder abuse within the Province of Québec. For our study this questionnaire underwent minor modifications in layout and content to assist the social workers in recording information in a way that would facilitate our research. While the resulting tool, the Social Worker Evaluation (SWE), was designed to aid the social workers in forming clinical impressions, it was not formally constructed to be a research tool. Nonetheless, it did have the ability to generate data relevant to an examination of the impact of gender. Just over 3/4 of the subjects who were asked the EASI also had the SWE administered to them. The remaining 1/4 did not get the SWE either because they could not make themselves available within the protocol designated three week follow-up period or because they decided not to participate further in the study. No differences were found however between these two groups when they were compared for mean age, gender, language spoken, living arrangements, education received, self-rated health, or mental and physical comportment scores on the SF-12. Of 661 subjects who did receive the SWE, the social workers indicated that they felt confident in the identification of elder abuse for 79 of them. In this context, the overall estimated prevalence of abuse was 12.0%; for females the rate was 13.6% (57/419), and for males the rate was 9.1% (22/242). For a variety of reasons, 242 of the original 905 study subjects who underwent the EASI assessment did not have a follow-up with the

SWE. Yet, the estimated prevalence for elder abuse from the SWE is remarkably similar to those cited above for the EASI.

Challenges in Gender Specificity Research

The SWE had the potential to record responses, for each individual, to personal, family, lifestyle, living conditions, relationship, health, and financial questions that the elder abuse literature has suggested may be related to abuse. Within the previously stated limits of the SWE as a research tool, responses were examined in an exploratory and descriptive way for those seniors identified as abused, with the objective of trying to generate some hypotheses of what might differentiate male and female victims. Once variables were eliminated because they did not appear to be proportionately different or cell counts would likely be low or absent in bivariate analyses, a Fisher's exact test was applied to the 15 remaining variables. Only one showed a statistically significant gender difference, and this could statistically be expected solely on the basis of the number of analyses performed. Specifically, abused males reported less participation in social activities than non-abused men ($p = 0.003$), an association not seen in women. This exercise highlights the need to have large samples of elder abuse victims in order to have sufficiently adequate sub-samples of males and females on whom to do more in-depth analyses.

SUMMARY

While family practice is an important setting in which to identify elder abuse, published reasons have been cited to explain why physician detection of such mistreatment is low. That literature has not explored the role that gender of either doctor or patient may play in identification of elder abuse. This paper has therefore explored other physician–patient contexts where a gender factor has appeared important and might extend to elder abuse. While some of these findings appear contradictory, extrapolation from them to the sensitive area of elder abuse suggests the possible role that gender bias may play, and supports the need for an objective tool such as the EASI for doctors to use. The implications of this are not inconsequential given the EASI development and validation findings that for every three older women identified as abused, there are two men also identified.

REFERENCES

Abuful, A., Gidron,Y., & Henkin,Y. (2005). Physicians' attitudes toward preventive therapy for coronary artery disease: Is there a gender bias? *Clinical Cardiology, 28,* 389-93.

Alter, D.A., Naylor, C.D., Austin, P.C., & Tu, J.V. (2002). Biology or bias: Practice patterns and long-term outcomes for men and women with acute myocardial infarction. *Journal of American College of Cardiology, 19,* 1909-1916.

Bertakis, K.L., Helms, L.J., Callahan, E.J., Azari, R., Leigh, P., & Robbins, J.A. (2001). Patient gender differences in the diagnoses of depression in primary care. *Journal of Women's Health & Gender–Based Medicine, 10,* 689-698.

Bloom, J.S., Ansel, P., & Bloom, M.N. (1989). Detecting elder abuse: A guide for physicians. *Geriatrics, 44,* 40-44.

Burd, I.D., Nevadunsky, N., & Bachmann, G.J. (2006). Impact of physician gender on sexual history taking in a multidisciplinary practice. *Journal of Sexual Medicine, 3,* 194-200.

Flocke, S.A., & Gilchrist, V. (2005). Physician and patient gender concordance and the delivery of comprehensive clinical preventive services. *Medical Care, 43,* 486-492.

Gabbard-Alley, A.S. (1995). Health communication and gender: A review and critique. *Health Communication, 7,* 35-54.

Gulbrandsen, P., Fugelli, P., & Hjortdahl, P. (1998). Psychosocial problems presented by patients with somatic reasons for encounter: Tip of the iceberg? *Family Practice, 15,* 1-8.

Gulbrandsen, P., Hjortdahl, P., & Fugelli, P. (1999). General practitioners' knowledge of their patients' psychosocial problems: Multipractice questionnaire survey. *British Medical Journal, 314,* 1014-1018.

Hall, J.A., Irish, J.T., Roter, D.L., Ehrlich, C.M., & Miller, H.L. (1994a) Gender in medical encounters: An analysis of physician and patient communication in a primary care setting. *Health Psychology, 13,* 384-392.

Hall, J.A., Irish, J.T., Roter, D.L., Ehrlich, C.M ., & Miller, H.L. (1994b). Satisfaction, gender, and communication in medical visits. *Medical Care, 32,* 1216-1231.

Hamberg, K., Risberg, G., Johansson, E.E., & Westman G. (2002). Gender bias in physicians' management of neck pain: A study of the answers in a Swedish national examination. *Journal of Women's Health and Gender Based Medicine, 11,* 653-666.

Harrell, R., Tornjo, C.H., McLaughlan, J., Pavlik, V.N., Hyman, D.J., & Dyer. C. (2002). How geriatricians identify elder abuse and neglect. *American Journal of the Medical Sciences, 323,* 34-38.

Henderson, J.T., & Weisman, C.S. (2001). Physician gender effects on preventive screening and counseling : An analysis of male and female patients' health care experiences. *Medical Care, 39,* 1281-1292.

Hendrix, K.H., Riehle, J.E., & Egan, B.M. (2005). Ethnic, gender, and age-related differences in treatment and control of dyslipidemia in hypertensive patients. *Ethnicity and Disease, 15,*11-16.

Hopman, W.M., Towheed, T., Anastassiades, T., Tenenhouse, A., Poliquin, S., Berger, C. et al. (2000). Canadian normative data for the SF-36 health survey. *Canadian Medical Association Journal, 163,* 265-271.

Jaglal, S.B., Slaughter, P.M., Baigrie, R.S., Morgan, C.D., & Naylor, C.D. (1995). Good judgment or sex bias in the referral of patients for the diagnosis of coronary artery disease? An exploratory study. *Canadian Medical Association Journal, 152*, 873-880.

Jones, J.S., Veensta, T.R., Seamon, J.P., & Krohmer, J. (1997). Elder mistreatment: A national survey of emergency physicians. *Annals of Emergency Medicine, 30*, 473-479.

Kennedy, R.D. (2005). Elder abuse and neglect: The experience, knowledge, and attitudes of primary care physicians. *Family Medicine, 37*, 81-5.

Kosberg, J.I. (2002). Heterosexual males: A group forgotten by the profession of social work. *Journal of Sociology and Social Welfare, 29*, 51-70.

Kosberg, J.I. (2005). Meeting the needs of older men: Challenges for those in helping professions. *Journal of Sociology and Social Welfare, 32*, 9-31.

Kozak, J.F., Elmslie, T., & Verdon, J. (1995). Epidemiological perspectives on the abuse and neglect of seniors: A review of the national and international literature. In M.J. Maclean (Ed.), *Abuse and neglect of older Canadians: Strategies for change* (pp. 129-139). Ottawa: Canadian Association of Gerontology and Toronto: Thompson Education Publishing.

Lachs, M.S., & Pillemer K. (2004). Elder abuse. *Lancet, 364*, 1263-1272.

McWhinney, I.R. (1989). *A textbook of family medicine.* Oxford: Oxford University Press.

Morabia, A., Fabre, J., & Dunand, J.P. (1992). The influence of patient and physician gender on prescription of psychotropic drugs. *Journal of Clinical Epidemiology, 45*, 111-116.

Mouton, C.P., Talamantes, M., Parker, R.W., Espino, D.V., & Miles, T.P. (2001). Abuse and neglect of older men. *Clinical Gerontologist, 24*, 15-26.

O'Brien, J.G. (1986) Elder abuse and the physician. *Michigan Medicine, 85*, 618-620.

O'Donnell, S.M. (2003). A comparison of physicians' verbal and non-verbal communication patterns with their younger and older patients. *Dissertation Abstract International: Section B: The Sciences and Engineerin, 63*(8-B).

Pritchard, J. (2001). *Male victims of elder abuse: Their experiences and needs.* London: Jessica Kingsley Publishers.

Raine, R.A., Crayford, T.J., Chan, K.L., & Chambers, J.B. (1999). Gender differences in the treatment of patients with acute myocardial ischemia and infarction in England. *International Journal of Technology Assessment in Health Care, 15*, 136-146.

Reiser, D.E., & Rosen, D.H. (1984). *Medicine as a human experience.* Baltimore: University Park Press.

Schulman, K.A., Berlin, J.A., Harless, W., Kerner, J.F., Sistrunk, S., Gersh, B.J. et al. (1999). The effect of race and sex on physicians' recommendations for cardiac catheterization. *New England Journal of Medicine, 340*, 618-626.

Shiels, C., & Gabby, M. (2006). The influence of GP and patient gender on the duration of certified sickness absence. *Family Practice, 23*, 246-252.

Sleuth, B., & Rubin, R.H. (2002). Gender, ethnicity, and physician–patient communication about depression and anxiety in primary care. *Patient Education and Counseling, 48*, 243-252.

Tomlin, S. (1988). *Abuse of elderly people: An unnecessary and preventable problem.* London: British Geriatrics Society.

Wolosin, R.J. (2005). The voice of the patient: A national representative study of satisfaction with family physicians. *Quality Management in Health Care,14*,155-164.

Yaffe, M.J., & Stewart, M.A. (1985). Factors influencing doctors' awareness of the life problems of middle aged patients. *Medical Care, 23*, 1276-1282.

Yaffe, M.J., Wolfson, C., Lithwick, M., & Weiss, D. (2006, October). The Elder Abuse Suspicion Index: A method to improve identification of elder abuse by doctors. *Proceedings of 34th North American Primary Care Research Group Annual Meeting.* Tuscon, AZ.

Young, J.M., & Ward, J.E. (1998). Influence of physician and patient gender on provision of smoking cessation advice in general practice. *Tobacco Control, 7*, 360-363.

Zaharias, G., Piterman, L., & Liddell, M. (2004). Doctors and patients: Gender interaction in the consultation. *Academic Medicine, 79*, 148-155.

Zlotnick, C., Elkin, I., & Shea, M.T. (1998). Does the gender of a patient or the gender of a therapist affect the treatment of patients with major depression. *Journal of Consultation Psychiatry, 66*, 655-659.

doi:10.1300/J084v19n01_04

Osteoporosis:
An Invisible, Undertreated,
and Neglected Disease of Elderly Men

Marilyn L. Haas, PhD, RN, CNS, ANP-C
Katen Moore, MSN, APRN, BC, AOCN®

SUMMARY. This article highlights a silent disease that threatens the health and vitality of older men. Among elderly men and women, osteoporosis is among one of the leading causes of morbidity and mortality in the United States. Once perceived as only a female dominated disease, osteoporosis is now known to be gender blind. The following discussion will review the epidemiology and pathology of osteoporosis, and identify the concerns raised for men, including neglect. Special management considerations for older men and recommendations for future research into this overlooked major health problem will be explored. Better understanding of how osteoporosis affects older men may help to encourage prevention strategies earlier in life, appropriate screening and monitoring, as well as more effective treatment later in life. doi:10.1300/J084v19n01_05 *[Article copies available for a fee from The Haworth Document Delivery Service: 1-800-HAWORTH. E-mail address: <docdelivery@haworthpress.com> Website: <http://www.HaworthPress.com> © 2007 by The Haworth Press, Inc. All rights reserved.]*

Marilyn L. Haas is a Nurse Practitioner, Mountain Radiation Oncology, Asheville, NC (E-mail: mlyhaas@worldnet.att.net). Katen Moore is a Nurse Practitioner, Radiation Oncology Service, NJHCS, Department of Veterans Affairs, East Orange, NJ (E-mail: katen.moore@med.va.gov).

[Haworth co-indexing entry note]: "Osteoporosis: An Invisible, Undertreated, and Neglected Disease of Elderly Men." Haas, Marilyn L., and Katen Moore. Co-published simultaneously in *Journal of Elder Abuse & Neglect*™ (The Haworth Maltreatment & Trauma Press®, an imprint of The Haworth Press, Inc.) Vol. 19, No. 1/2, 2007, pp. 61-73; and: *Abuse of Older Men* (ed: Jordan I. Kosberg) The Haworth Maltreatment & Trauma Press®, an imprint of The Haworth Press, Inc., 2007, pp. 61-73. Single or multiple copies of this article are available for a fee from The Haworth Document Delivery Service [1-800-HAWORTH, 9:00 a.m. - 5:00 p.m. (EST). E-mail address: docdelivery@haworthpress.com].

KEYWORDS. Osteoporosis, bone density, fragility fractures, male gender, risk indicators, screening prevention

INTRODUCTION

The National Institutes of Health consensus panel, chaired by Dr. Anne Klibanski in 2000, describes osteoporosis as "a skeletal disorder characterized by compromised bone strength predisposing a person to an increased risk of fracture" (National Consensus Development Panel on Osteoporosis, Prevention, Diagnosis, and Therapy, 2001, p. 786). To date, most research and clinical studies have focused on this disease in women. One of the largest studies, the National Osteoporosis Risk Assessment (NORA) which began in 1997, excluded men intentionally focusing only on postmenopausal women. Yet, osteoporosis is a major health threat to men as well. While osteoporosis is certainly less prevalent in men than women, the diagnosis still affects about 3.5 million men in the United States, with 1.5 million men over 65 at risk (Finkelstein, 2006). Bone fractures in particular are the major complication from osteoporosis and the incidence of hip fracture is thirty percent greater in older men than older women (Kenny, Prestwood, Marcello, & Raisz, 2000). It is important to note that the mortality rate for men following hip fractures surpasses that of women.

It is the purpose of this article to suggest that the inattention to the possibility of osteoporosis for men can be considered an example of neglectful behavior. There is evidence of both the existence of such problems for men as well as the under-diagnosis of the problem within the health care field. The inability to advocate for periodic detection of the problem for older men can result in health problems that are associated with social, psychological, physical, and economic consequences. To be discussed will be the problem of osteoporosis, risk factors for older men, need for specific diagnosis guidelines for men, and effective treatment modalities that can be used with them. The article concludes with suggestions for needed efforts that result in greater understanding of the causes of this health problem that affects older men and needed interventions that focus on both effective prevention and treatment interventions.

Osteoporosis can have physical, financial, and psychosocial effects, all of which have a direct impact on the quality of life for that person along with the family and community. Acute pain from fractures can lead to chronic pain. Chronic pain has its own associated costs and can be debilitating over time. Also, chronic pain decreases personal and/or social activities. Capturing only the direct financial expenditures for the treatment of osteoporotic fractures is estimated to be between 10-15 billion dollars annually (NIH Consensus Development Panel on Osteoporosis, Prevention, Diagnosis, and Therapy, 2001). These figures do not take into account the indirect costs of fracture, such as loss of time from employment, disability or unemployment. Finally, fractures can lead to the loss of physical independence and, from there, a host of psychosocial problems (i.e., depression, fear and/or anxiety, and changes in usual role function).

PATHOPHYSIOLOGY OF BONE LOSS

Bone mineral density (BMD) is a measurement of the level of minerals in the bones, which designates how dense and strong the bones are within the body. BMD estimates the true mass of the bone. Therefore BMD correlates to bone strength and its ability to bear weight.

All individuals begin losing bone mass after they reach peak BMD which is around age 30 (Orwoll, Oviatt, McClung et al., 1990). However, the thicker a person's bones are at age 30, the longer it will take to develop bone loss, and men generally have denser bones than women.

For any individual, healthy bone structure goes through a continuous process of resorption, which is bone breakdown, and formation. Certain cells called *osteoclasts* bind to the surface of the bone and break it down. Other bone forming cells referred to as *osteoblasts* then move in and help form new bone. This process occurs continuously in early life. However, in older age, bone formation fails to keep pace with resorption. The remodeling cycle begins to go out of balance. Men, along with women, experience an age-related decline in this process and BMD.

BMD that is lower than the normal peak BMD, but not low enough to be classified as osteoporosis, is referred to as osteopenia. Osteopenia is often viewed as a precursor to osteoporosis. Osteoporosis is a more serious condition that causes bones to become brittle and possibly break. Osteopenia does not have a specific symptom, such as pain, but can cause changes in stature and posture that evolve over time and is less recognizable to the clinician in a single encounter. For this reason, osteopenia is a silent process and an invisible disease that can quickly progress to osteoporosis. If this occurs, bones become less dense to the point that a fragility fracture can occur.

OSTEOPOROSIS RISK FACTORS FOR MEN

Numerous medical conditions, disease processes, or treatments are associated with men's risk of developing osteoporosis. The most common medical disorder is hypogonadism, where there is a reduction in the gonadal hormones (Kiebzak, Beinart, Perser, Ambrose, Siff, & Heggeness, 2003). This can be caused by congenital abnormalities or acquired diseases. For older men in particular, the cause may be associated with advanced prostate cancer where the treatment frequently includes androgen suppressive therapy to induce hypogonadism (i.e., orchiectomy, hormonal ablation, and chemotherapy). This reduction in hormones ultimately results in increased bone turnover, bone loss, and diminished bone strength (Daniell, Dunn, Ferguson, Lomas, Niazi, & Stratte, 2000).

Other factors that can contribute to developing osteoporosis for men include eating disorders, metabolic problems that do not allow proper absorption of vitamins and minerals, long term use of steroids to treat conditions such as asthma, autoimmune diseases, cancers, or exposure to radiation (Gholz, Conde, & Rutledge, 2002; Brinkley, Schmeer, Wasnich, & Lenchik, 2002). Reversible factors that can be determinants for bone loss for men are related to environmental factors and physical inactivity. Years of smoking, poor diet, excessive alcohol intake and low rates of physical activity also have been associated with increased rates of bone loss (Slemenda, Christian, Reed, Reiser, Williams, & Johnson, 1992; Kaufman, Jonell, Abadie et al., 2000).

MEASUREMENT TOOLS

The goal for preventing osteoporosis is to evaluate the risk of development, as well as to make recommendations for prevention. Simple physical assessments, such as measuring a man's height over time for comparison for loss of bone structure and posture assessment, are not being done by many healthcare providers and are not even considered for men's screening. Both of these assessments must become a routine part of the physical examination process during healthcare visits. Laboratory evaluations for secondary causes of osteoporosis for men also should be considered by healthcare clinicians when osteoporosis is diagnosed.

Currently, there are no accurate measurements for overall bone health and strength (see Table 1). Regular x-rays cannot detect mild bone loss, as the bone needs to lose at least a quarter of the density before

TABLE 1. Bone Assessment Measurements

Diagnostic Measurement	What's Being Measured
Bone Mineral Density–values taken from hip, spine, forearm, hand, heel	Bone mass Mineralization Bone density
Bone Turn Over–bone resorption and bone formation (bone remodeling)	Biochemical markers (urine and blood) e.g., blood levels of alkaline phosphatase and osteocalcin and urine levels of pyridinolines and deoxypyridinolines
Bone Quality–high resolution of MRI	Structure, porosity, and connectivity
Bone Quality–bone biopsies	Bone tissue for abnormalities

osteoporosis can be detected. Therefore, bone mineral density (BMD) is the closest measure of bone strength. The bone density test is a dual-energy x-ray absorptiometry, or commonly referred to as the DEXA scan. There are other tests, including computed tomography (CT) scans, dual photon asorptiometry (DPA) and ultrasound, but DEXA is by far the most prevalent in community practice. DEXA is also the device used by the World Health Organization (WHO) to determine the accepted diagnostic criteria for osteoporosis. It is very important that the same actual machine be used for serial DEXA scans as there is no machine to measure standardization. More alarming for healthcare clinicians and men is the T and Z-scores from the DEXA scans only represent standard deviations for young Caucasian adult women of northern European extraction. Scores are not representative of young or elderly men, nor do they represent a measure across ethnic groups (El-Hajj Fuleihan, Baddoura et al., 2002; Faulkner & Orwoll, 2002). This creates confusion for researchers, healthcare providers, and individual men themselves as they try to understand their individual risk, comparison to others, and treatment recommendations. Other assessments, but not generally utilized in screening, are magnetic resonance imaging (MRI) and bone biopsies.

ACCURATE DIAGNOSIS IN MEN

The WHO published diagnosis guidelines for osteoporosis, but again the standards are based on clinical trials among postmenopausal women. In 2003, the International Society for Clinical Densitometry (ISCD) recognized this fact and conducted a conference on osteoporosis and included the implications for men as well as those for premenopausal women and children. After this conference, the ISCD adopted guidelines for diagnosing osteoporosis in men who were 20 years of age and older (see Table 2). After reviewing and carefully considering the WHO's classifications, the ISCD recommends that WHO classifications should not be applied in its entirety to men. For men under 50 years of age, ISCD urges that diagnosis should not be made on the basis of densitometric criteria alone. Furthermore, men at any age with secondary causes of low BMD (e.g., glucocorticoid therapy, hypogonadism, and hyperparathyroidism) may be diagnosed clinically with osteoporosis supported by findings of low BMD, but have different fracture risk at a given BMD than healthy older men (Writing Group for the ISCD Position Development, 2004). Now older men, along with their healthcare clinicians, can diagnose osteoporosis that has a male reference database.

EFFECTIVE MEDICAL TREATMENTS

It was once believed that if an elderly person developed osteoporosis, medicine did not have anything to offer to rebuild the structure of the bones. However, scientific understanding of human aging has improved. Along with newer pharmaceutical discoveries, medicine can now offer more insight into the prevention and treatment of osteoporosis. Since most of the studies are still largely conducted on western Caucasian women (El-Hajj, Fuleihan, Baddoura et al., 2002), these interventions' effectiveness in men is extrapolated from limited data.

Non-Pharmacological Interventions

It is very important to monitor all men, not just women, to assess their risks for falls and provide appropriate intervention strategies to prevent falls and minimize fracture potentials. Balance exercises such as Tai Chi

TABLE 2. International Society for Clinical Densitometry Osteoporosis Diagnosis for Men

Age	Results Reported In T-Score Measurements
50-65 years old	T-scores (*may be used*) of –2.5 or less along with risk factors[*]
65 years and older	T-scores (*should be used*) of –2.5 or less[*]

[*]male reference database (Adapted from Writing Group for the ISCD Position Development Conference, 2004).

have been shown to be very successful in reducing the risk of falls by improving balance and recovery even in the very frail elderly (Wolf, Barnhart, Kutner et al., 1996). Weight bearing exercise is recommended with weight training to increase and maintain muscle strength and balance (Kaufman et al., 2000).

Calcium Supplemental Intervention

All older adult men who are at risk for bone density loss, or have a diagnosis of osteopenia or osteoporosis, should be taking an oral calcium/vitamin D supplement, unless contraindicated. Taking this supplement will not prevent, but may help retard, the progression of bone loss. While recommended doses vary from guideline to guideline, adequate intake is between 800-1800 mg calcium per day along with 400-800 IU per day of vitamin D, which helps absorption of the calcium (Epocrates, 2006). Exposure to direct sunlight ten to fifteen minutes, three times a week, also allows the body to manufacture adequate levels of vitamin D (Grossman & MacLean, 2001). These doses have not shown an effect on prostate cancer progression (Smith, 2003).

Taking higher doses of calcium may pose concerns. There are some reports that high dietary intake of calcium (>2000 mg daily) can increase risk of prostate cancer. While there is no evidence to prove a causal relationship between calcium intake and prostate cancer, there is currently concern for those men with high intakes of calcium enriched foods developing prostate cancer.

Pharmacological Interventions

Pharmaceutical interventions can be a considered to treat osteopenia or osteoporosis. The only osteoporosis treatments approved by the FDA for use in men are oral bisphosphonates, alendronate (Fosamax®, Merck, NJ) and risedronate (Actonel®, Proctor and Gamble). These drugs, taken for a total of five years, have shown to increase bone density in the vertebral spine and femoral neck. However, these drugs should not be taken by those with a history of gastric ulcer or gastrointestinal bleeding (Jan & Kaul, 2006). The oral bisphosphonates are usually taken once a week. Men should take the tablet first thing in the morning and remain fasting for one hour after taking. The tablet is taken with a full eight ounce glass of water only and the person taking it should remain standing or sitting upright for at least 30 minutes afterwards to prevent erosion of the lower esophagus.

Calcitonin (Miacalcin®, Novartis, New Jersey) is an old mainstay utilized for osteoporosis therapy. Unfortunately this medication has shown an insignificant effect on fracture risk reduction, thus should not be recommended for first line therapy in osteoporosis. Adherence rates are also poor with this medication, even though it is available as a nasal spray, or subcutaneous or intramuscular injection (Jan & Kaul, 2006).

Teriparatide (Forteo®, Eli Lilly, NJ), a parathyroid hormone (PTH) analogue, can be used in men with hypogonadal or idiopathic osteoporosis. It is injected daily for two years maximum. Teriparatide activates *osteoblastic* activity, increasing bone mass, formation and density similarly to PTH. It is contraindictated (black box warning in drug labeling) with Paget's disease due to concerns of increased risk of osteosarcoma (Jan & Kaul, 2006).

Testosterone replacement therapy is controversial in osteoporosis therapy, but has shown to be effective on bone density. However, it should not be used by men with normal gonadal function. Unfortunately, these are most of the men with osteoporosis. Men with hypogonadism are recommended by the American College of Rheumatology to consider testosterone therapy with T-score of more than −1.0 (Grossman & MacLean, 2001; Ringe, Faber & Dorst, 2001). Testosterone comes in different routes of administration and in various dosages. The clinician needs to decide which method of administration and how much of the drug to administer. Testosterone is produced by many pharmaceutical manufacturers, and is considered a schedule III controlled drug when prescribing and may not even be available to many prescribers.

Other Options for Off-Label Pharmaceutical Treatments

Sometimes the above pharmaceutical options are ineffective in men and other options need to be explored. It is important for any healthcare clinician to inform men when they are recommending off-label pharmaceutical interventions. An example of another oral bisphosphonates approved for osteoporosis treatment for women is Ibandronate (Boniva®, Roche, NJ). The efficacy in men is uncertain. Intravenous bisphosphonates can be given when oral bisphosphonates are contraindicated. Since the medication is given through the veins, it bypasses the esophagus, stomach and gut avoiding gastric irritation. The intravenous bisphosphonates include Pamidronate (Aredia®, Novartis, NJ), etidronate (Didronel®, Procter and Gamble) and zolendronic acid (Zometa®, Novartis, NJ). However, these drugs are not approved as primary treatments for osteoporosis in men. All bisphosphonates (oral and intravenous) have been linked with osteonecrosis, a serious adverse effect in the jawbone (Ruggiero, Mehrotra, Rosenberg, & Engroff, 2004). Therefore, it is extremely important for men who are taking this medication to be taught to report *any* pain in the jaw or mouth immediately to a dental or healthcare professional. It is also recommended that the prescriber contact the patient's dentist to report the initiation of bisphosphonate therapy (Ruggiero, Mehrotra, Rosenberg, & Engroff).

DIRECTION FOR FUTURE RESEARCH

Osteoporosis is a major medical and public health problem for the elderly. While bone loss is prevalent among both men and women, there needs to be more epidemiological studies that involve aging men. There are numerous potential factors that can influence how men lose BMD. Before effective treatment can be recommended, the underlying etiology in men needs to be better understood and researched. Interventional studies need to include more men in order to make evidence-based recommendations. Recently, it was reported that a protein structure in the body was easily manipulated to increase bone mass in mice. Humans share this same protein and may benefit from this research in the future if the manipulation successfully balances the *osteoclast/osteoblast* ratio closer to that of younger adulthood (Yeo, McDonald, & Zayzafoon, 2006). Hopefully, a study like this and others would need to include an equal ratio of men and women, young and old. Interventional studies also should include equal ratios of men and women of varied ethnic and racial backgrounds, so society will benefit as a whole in decreasing this disease.

Osteoporosis should be treated as a major potential debilitating disease of all aging adults, including men. Research with prevention would, of course, be more prudent than treating osteoporosis complications in later life. Screening and subsequent appropriate management of individuals with early signs of bone density loss should be just as common as other diagnostic tests for men (e.g., PSA blood screening for prostate cancer or colonoscopy for screening for colon cancer). Prevention and screening for osteoporosis is generally overlooked in men; therefore, it often goes unrecognized or is not treated as aggressively. Emphasis should be given equally to gender-sensitive intervention recommendations. This cannot be done unless there are more clinical studies involving aging men.

Studies are needed to understand the role of cost-effective measures, too (e.g., dietary supplements, nutritional or cultural influences, and genetics).

Special considerations and assessments should focus on elderly men who have cancer and were given androgen ablation treatments to help cure or control their cancer, along with other aging ailments and diseases. Prevention research strategies could include education about aging and the impact of poor dietary habits, poor physical functioning with lack of exercise, excessive alcohol intake, or tobacco abuse. These all have deleterious effects on achieving bone mass and maintaining it during later life. Also, risk fracture assessment tools, administered by healthcare clinicians, could bring this disease forward in the minds of the elderly men to make lifestyle changes at home or in long-term care facilities and stress the importance of medication regimes.

While osteoporosis is not a new problem, it is still in its infancy in regards to men overall, and more evidence-based studies are needed to protect men from the hidden dangers of this disease. While scientists may never discover a way to halt or reverse this disease, it is never too late to begin lifestyle changes that can help stop the progression of osteoporosis. Regular exercise, well-balanced meals, smoking cessation, and avoiding excessive alcohol intake can all retard the process of bone loss, delay osteopenia, or prevent osteoporosis. Keeping regular health examinations will help both men and their healthcare clinicians decide the best appropriate interventions to combat this preventable, yet under diagnosed, disease among men.

CONCLUSIONS

There are health disparities between elderly men and women. Osteoporosis is one example that depicts this inequality. While men are socialized to think they are invincible early in life, which can carry over into adulthood, men's bodies undergo physiological changes that require attention in later years. Men need to learn how to become proactive in their healthcare and should seek out screening measures, e.g., bone density testing, along with other standard screening for the prostate and colorectal cancers.

This responsibility can begin with men learning more about osteoporosis and their risk factors. This can be accomplished by engaging in educational community activities. Informative educational presentations are given by volunteer civic organizations (e.g., Rotarians, Kiwanis, or Civitan Clubs), church men's groups, mall screenings, barber shops, or exercise gymnasiums (e.g., YMCA). All of these informal settings can provide opportunities for education and screening. Early detection can help with interventions that could prevent fractures later in life.

Besides community support, healthcare providers also need to place similar emphasis on annual screening for men beyond the routine prostate and colorectal screening. This can begin in educational classes for medical and nursing students, requiring geriatric issues integrated in curriculums. Distinctions between elderly men and women should be presented. Once in practice, all specialties should be mindful of prevention and lifestyle behaviors of men. Urologists should be just as diligent as primary care physicians in inquiring about all male-related screening tests, as their appointments maybe the only visits men seek a year. Both non-pharmaceutical and pharmaceutical interventions should be recommended as early as possible.

Fortunately, those men who do seek medical care regarding osteoporosis screening and medical care will find that osteoporosis is a reimbursable diagnosis and therefore covered by many private insurance companies and Medicare (http://www.gehealthcare.com/usen/community/reimbursement/docs/BoneDensityAdvisory.pdf). Men can seek specialized care through ambulatory clinics designed to care for men diagnosed with osteoporosis. It is encouraging that more clinics are opening and being developed, thus placing emphasis on this disease. With more concentrated efforts on this disease, osteoporosis in men can be prevented or managed early to prevent fractures later.

Thus, there are increasing efforts to systematically screen and detect osteoporosis in older men, along with efforts to use protocols that have been standardized on them. In such efforts, the medical and nursing community will reflect equitable concern for this "silent disease" in men as well as in women. As with any other type of health care problem that affects both sexes, discrepancies in the concern, assessment, and intervention of one rather than for both can be considered neglectful medical care. It is hoped that this article will underscore the need for greater attention to be given to men and, thus, result in more equitable and effective care for both men and women.

REFERENCES

Brinkley, N., Schmeer, P., Wasnich, R., & Lenchik, L. (2002). What are the criteria by which a densitometric diagnosis of osteoporosis can be made in males and non-Caucasians? *Journal of Clinical Densitometry, 5*, suppl, S19-27.

Daniell, H., Dunn, S., Ferguson, D., Lomas, G., Niazi, Z., & Stratte, P. (2000). Progressive osteoporosis during androgen deprivation therapy for prostate cancer. *Journal of Urology, 163*, 181-186.

El-Hajj, G., Fuleihan, G., Baddoura, R., Awada, H., Okais, J., Rizk, P., & McClung, M. (2002). Practice guidelines on the use of bone mineral density measurements: Who to test? What measures to use? When to treat?: A consensus report from the Middle East Densitometry Workshop. *Lebanese Medical Journal, 50*(3), 89-104.

Epocrates Rx [database for PDA]. Version 7.50. San Mateo (CA): Epocrates, Inc., 1999–[updated 2006 Nov 2; cited 2006 Nov 2]. Available from: http://www.epocrates.com. Drug information for Palm OS or Microsoft Pocket PC handheld devices; content updates via Hot Sync.

Faulkner, K., & Orwoll, E. (2002). Implications in the use of T-scores for the diagnosis of osteoporosis in men. *Journal Clinical Densitometry, 5*(1), 87-93.

Finkelstein, J. (2006). Overview of osteoporosis in men, Up-to-date. http://www.utdol.com/utd/content/topic.do?topicKey=minmetab/20928&view=text

Gholz, R., Conde, R., & Rutledge, D. (2002). Osteoporosis in men treated with androgen suppression therapy for prostate cancer. *Clinical Journal of Oncology Nursing, 6*(2), 88-93.

Grossman, J., & MacLean, C. (2001). Quality indicators for the management of osteoporosis in vulnerable elders. *Annals of Internal Medicine, 135*(8, part 2), 722-730.

Jan, S., & Kaul, A. (2006). Osteoporosis: Prevention and treatment. *Journal of Managed Care Medicine, 9*(1), 11-21.

Kaufman, J., Jonell, O., Abadie, E., Adami, S., Audran, M., Avouac, B. et al. (2000). Background for studies on the treatment of male osteoporosis: State of the art. *Annals of Rheumatologic Disease, 59*, 765-772.

Kenny, A., Prestwood, K., Marcello, K., & Raisz, L. (2000). Determinants of bone density in healthy older men with low testosterone levels. *Journal of Gerontology A: Biological Science/Medical Science, 55*, 492-497.

Kiebzak, A., Beinart, K., Perser, C., Ambrose, K., Siff, S., & Heggeness, M. (2003). Hypogonadism and osteoporosis in men. *Archives of Internal Medicine. 163*, 1237-1238.

National Consensus Development Panel on Osteoporosis Prevention, Diagnosis, and Therapy. (2001). Osteoporosis prevention, diagnosis, and therapy. *Journal of the American Medical Association, 285*(6), 785-795.

Orwoll, E., Oviatt, S., McClung, M. et al. (1990). The rate of bone mineral loss in normal men and the effects of calcium and cholecalciferol supplementation. *Annals of Internal Medicine, 112*, 29.

Ringe, J., Faber, H., & Dorst, A. (2001). Alendronate treatment of established primary osteoporosis in men: Results of a 2 year prospective study. *Journal of Clinical Endocrinology & Metabolism, 86*(11), 5252-5255.

Ruggiero, S., Mehrotra, B., Rosenberg, T., & Engroff, S. (2004). Osteonecrosis of the jaws associated with the use of bisphosphonates: A review of 63 cases. *Journal of Oral Maxillofacial Surgery, 62*(5), 527-34.

Slemenda, C., Christain, J., Reed, T., Reister, T., William, C., & Johnston, C. (1992). Long-term bone loss in men: Effects of genetic and environmental factors. *Annals of Internal Medicine, 117*(4), 286-291.

Smith, M. (2003). Diagnosis and management of treatment-related osteoporosis in men with prostate carcinoma. *Cancer: Skeletal complications of malignancy supplement, 97*(3), 789-795.

Wolf, S. Barnhart, H., Kutner, N., McNeely, E., Coogler, C., & Xu, T. (1996). Reducing fraity and falls in older persons: An investigation of Tai Chi and computerized balance training. Atlanta FICSIT Group. Frailty and Injuries: Cooperative Studies of Intervention Techniques. *Journal of the American Geriatric Society, 44*(5), 489-497.

Writing Group for the ISCD Position Development Conference. 2004, Diagnosis of osteoporosis in men, premenopausal women, and children. *Journal of Clinical Densitometry, 7*(1), 17-26.

Yeo, H., McDonald, J., & Zayzafoon, M. (2006). NFATc1: A novel anabolic therapeutic target for osteoporosis. *Annals of the New York Academy of Sciences, 1068*, 564.

doi:10.1300/J084v19n01_05

Fractured Relationships
and the Potential for Abuse of Older Men

Dorothy C. Stratton, MSW, ACSW
Alinde J. Moore, PhD

SUMMARY. Elderly men are an understudied population in the area of abuse and neglect. The typical elder abuse or neglect victim is described as a frail woman. The National Elder Abuse Incidence Study shows men to be victims as well and at higher risk than women for abandonment, the most extreme form of neglect. A qualitative study of older widowed men did not specifically explore issues of abuse and neglect, but found several of the men experiencing alienation from one or more of their adult children. This paper explores the dynamics of these "fractured relationships" and finds several patterns that may increase an older man's risk of being neglected when his needs for support increase. Many men are not functioning in a kinkeeper role and are not attempting to repair fractured relationships. Minimizing their own feelings may prevent men from understanding the extent of alienation felt by an adult child. doi:10.1300/J084v19n01_06 *[Article copies available for a fee from The Haworth Document Delivery Service: 1-800-HAWORTH. E-mail address: <docdelivery@haworthpress.com> Website: <http://www.HaworthPress.com> © 2007 by The Haworth Press, Inc. All rights reserved.]*

Dorthy C. Stratton is associated with Ashland University, Department of Social Work, 401 College Avenue, Ashland, OH 44805 (E-mail: dstratto@ashland.edu). Alinde J. Moore is associated with Ashland University, Department of Psychology, 401 College Avenue, Ashland, OH 44805 (E-mail: amoore@ashland.edu).

[Haworth co-indexing entry note]: "Fractured Relationships and the Potential for Abuse of Older Men." Stratton, Dorothy C., and Alinde J. Moore. Co-published simultaneously in *Journal of Elder Abuse & Neglect*™ (The Haworth Maltreatment & Trauma Press®, an imprint of The Haworth Press, Inc.) Vol. 19, No. 1/2, 2007, pp. 75-97; and: *Abuse of Older Men* (ed: Jordan I. Kosberg) The Haworth Maltreatment & Trauma Press®, an imprint of The Haworth Press, Inc., 2007, pp. 75-97. Single or multiple copies of this article are available for a fee from The Haworth Document Delivery Service [1-800-HAWORTH, 9:00 a.m. - 5:00 p.m. (EST). E-mail address: docdelivery@haworthpress.com].

KEYWORDS. Older widowers, adult children, elder neglect, men's relationships, alienation

INTRODUCTION

The potential for victimization of elderly men by family members is beginning to draw research attention. Women are more often victimized, but they are not the only victims. The *National Elder Abuse Incidence Study* (National Center on Elder Abuse, 1998) found that elderly men are subject to mistreatment in all categories of abuse and neglect and are more likely than women to be victims of abandonment, the conscious rejection of responsibility to provide care.

BACKGROUND

A qualitative study of 51 older men (Moore & Stratton, 2002) was based upon the grounded theory of Glaser and Strauss (1967). The purpose of the study was to identify characteristics and behaviors that led some men to make satisfactory adjustment of life after the loss of a spouse; the themes and patterns of the men who seemed to have adjusted well were of particular interest. The purposive sample was located through a network of professional and personal acquaintances who first contacted the participants. The participants ranged in age from 58 to 104 years, averaging 80 years. They lived in various states of the United States and in provinces in Canada. All were widowed; four had lost more than one wife. Fourteen had remarried, and three more married after the interviews. The men were interviewed concerning their life with their spouses and subsequent adjustment to loss, and the interviews were conducted on two different days with follow-up telephone interviews for most of the men. Tape-recorded interviews were transcribed verbatim and coded for categories, topics, and themes. A general finding was that most men were coping with the loss in a way that allowed them to regain meaning and a sense of satisfaction with life, although the individual coping strategies varied greatly.

We did not interview our men about abuse; yet, the topic emerged in discussions. For example, Jim said his wife had become angry with him in the car on the way home from the grocery store one day and had hit him in the head with a loaf of bread while he was driving. Craig said his wife hit him with a lamp once in an angry outburst. These were presented to us as isolated incidents, and they were the only reports of physical violence victimization in the marital relationships of our respondents.

Most of them were currently living alone or with new wives. Only four of the 51 widowed men we interviewed lived with an adult child; all of those men were very old (ages 83-100). We interviewed the men in their homes and met their caregivers. The men were being well cared for; there were no signs of elder abuse or neglect in these households. However, one of the men had been controlling and harsh with both his wife and his son. His situation led us to wonder how and why his son treated him so well, as if we expected neglect or abuse would be the "normal" response to treatment such as the son had received from his father and had witnessed his mother receiving.

Also, we saw a pattern in the relationships of some men with their adult children that we characterized as alienation (Moore & Stratton, 2002), which represented conflict or disagreement that had led to a minimizing of contact. Cicirelli (1986) describes one way of dealing with conflict as mutual withdrawal. Nydegger and Mitteness (1991) observed fathers and adult children limiting contact to avoid conflict. This seemed to be the most common way our respondents were dealing with the children with whom they were in conflict. Yet we were interviewing these men (mean age 80) at a time when some dependence on others was necessary or would soon be necessary. If these men had fractured relationships with their children, what would be the chances for neglect or abandonment of the elder father when he was in need?

Having noted a theme of alienation from an adult child for several of the men, we then identified several patterns within those cases:

> (a) a child was viewed as immature or irresponsible and mother was blamed for having coddled the child, (b) the father disliked a child's spouse, (c) the father had strong opinions and expressed little tolerance for someone who did not live up to expectations, (d) an adult child had negative feelings about the widowed father's new intimate relationship, (e) the father was not actively trying to resolve the alienation, and (f) all children were not equally alienated from the father. (Moore & Stratton, 2002, p. 187)

Fractured relationships seemed to stem from early harsh or emotionally distant fathering, personality clashes and/or conflicts involving the father criticizing the child, or a child not able to accept the widowed father's repartnering. We also observed that the fathers were not making much effort to improve their fractured relationships. Thus, we became

interested in the nature and course of conflicted father/child relationships
that had the potential to become abusive or neglectful. In this article we
also will consider dynamics that moderate that risk.

THE PROBLEM

Definitions and Descriptions of Abuse, Neglect, and Abandonment

A cultural context of ageism in America, in which older persons are
devalued by themselves and by others, sets the stage for mistreatment
and acceptance of mistreatment (Butler, 1969; Kosberg & Nahmiash,
1996). Isolation is the hallmark of elder abuse and neglect, much more
than of child mistreatment. No teacher or coach will observe and become suspicious of bruises, weight loss, or timid withdrawn behavior.
The isolation of elder victims contributes to their invisibility in society
(Kosberg, 1998) and therefore to the under-reporting of abuse and neglect
cases (National Center on Elder Abuse, 1998).

Definitions of abuse, neglect, and abandonment are not uniform across
jurisdictions or among researchers, but the mistreatment suffered by
some elders can be broadly characterized under these categories: physical abuse, sexual abuse, emotional or psychological abuse, material or
financial abuse, and neglect (National Center on Elder Abuse, 1998;
Whittaker, 1996; Wolf, 1996). Neglect involves an act or a failure or re-
fusal to act (by a person with an obligation to help) that puts the safety
and well-being of a dependent person at risk. Self-neglect occurs when
a person living alone is not able to provide adequately for his or her own
safety and health. Self-neglect represents more than half of the cases
substantiated by Adult Protective Services (Tatara, 1993). It often occurs because family members are not tending to the circumstances and
needs of the elder person. Neglect can be active or passive, depending
upon the intention of the perpetrator to cause harm (Cicirelli, 1986). Financial abuse can result in neglect when the elder person suffers for
want of something that could have been purchased if his or her funds
had not been misappropriated. Abandonment amounts to desertion and
is the conscious rejection of responsibility to provide care for a person
when a legal or moral obligation to do so exists. As such, abandonment
is an extreme form of active neglect.

The *National Elder Abuse Incidence Study* (National Center on Elder
Abuse, 1998) funded by the federal government, is the source for recent
statistics on elder abuse and neglect. The study found nearly 450,000

persons aged 60 and older were abused or neglected in their home setting. Another 101,000 were self-neglecting. Only 21% of these cases had been reported to Adult Protective Services and substantiated. Neglect by a caregiver represented nearly half of the substantiated cases of maltreatment, with ages 80 and older at the highest risk. While most studies of elder abuse show more women as victims, the victimization of men also has received attention (Kosberg, 1998; Pillemer & Finkelhor, 1988; Tatara, 1993; Whittaker, 1996). Elderly men, especially those who are frail, can be victims of abuse by both male and female perpetrators (Pillemer & Wolf, 1986). Kosberg noted that men are more likely to self-abuse, particularly with alcohol, and thus may set themselves up to be more vulnerable to others. Also, they may use alcohol to escape the distress of abuse or neglect. According to Pritchard (2001), abused men are not likely to disclose their situation. Steinmetz (1977-78) described and analyzed husband-battering, describing it as "not uncommon," "hidden under a cloak of secrecy," and an "example of selective inattention" (p. 499). The *National Elder Abuse Incidence Study* shows men to be at higher risk than women for abandonment, with persons ages 75-79 at the highest risk. Adult children (47%) form the largest category of perpetrators.

Factors that could contribute to neglect potential have been identified by many researchers. In a review of the literature on elder abuse and neglect, Kosberg and Nahmiash (1996) identify characteristics of elderly victims, their abusers, and the social and cultural context within which the abuse or neglect occurs. Early descriptions of elder abuse situations highlighted the frailty and dependency of the elder, but that is not always the case. Adult children who neglect or abuse are often financially dependent upon their elder parent and have mental health or substance abuse problems (Greenberg & Becker, 1988; Kosberg & Nahmiash; Pillemer & Finkelhor, 1989; Wolf, 1996).

The Illinois Risk Assessment Protocol, as presented by Hwalek, Goodrich, and Quinn (1996), adds the issue of control and perpetrator/victim dynamics that can contribute to risk of abuse and neglect. Kosberg and Nahmiash (1996) further identify contributing social contexts, including financial problems of the caregiver, a history of family violence, family disharmony, lack of social support, and living arrangements. These authors maintain that mistreatment occurs within a milieu of cultural norms that include ageism, sexism, attitudes about violence, reactions to abuse, attitudes about disabilities, and family caregiving beliefs.

This article is limited to a consideration of the father-child relationship dynamics that have the potential risk of becoming situations of neglect. We will define neglect through examples of scenarios that we could envision unfolding in the lives of our widowed respondents as they lose their ability to live independently. Such possibilities include contacting the father very infrequently (even by telephone), not including the father in family events and activities, not engaging the father in sincere and interested interaction, not having regard for the father's loneliness, failing to see that the father gets needed medical care, failing to provide adequately for the father's comfort or failing to arrange for household assistance, and misusing the father's resources. Abandonment would involve not having contact at all with the father, nor taking any responsibility to be informed about his circumstances–much less do anything about them.

POSSIBLE ANTECDENTS FOR RELATIONSHIP FRACTURES

Personalities/Characteristics of the Men

Taking care not to adopt a deficit model for viewing older men overall (Boxer, Cook, & Cohler, 1986), as many men have very positive family relationships, we do see patterns that are quite common for men which have the potential for increasing relationship fractures and thereby decreasing the likelihood of family support in old age. Such possible patterns include the following: Some men tend to refrain from kinkeeping, minimize their feelings and problems, do not seek help, do not try to repair their fractured relationships, and/or have a personality style of negativity that makes most or all relationships difficult.

Kinkeeping. Hagestad (1986) identifies women as the ones who keep in contact with family members and arrange family activities. Many of our respondents described their wives (and some their new wives) as taking on that kinkeeping role (Moore & Stratton, 2002). Why do not more men take on such a role? Is it because they do not know how? Because they are not allowed to by the womenfolk? Because they are indifferent to family relations? There were exceptional men at kinkeeping, but our respondent Garrett was more representative. He had to call in his second wife to recall the ages and birth dates of his own children. Kinkeeping is considered in greater depth later in the section on contact and quality in the father-child relationship.

Masculine minimizing. In the Pillemer & Finkelhor study (1988), male victims reported less severe abuse and less emotional upset than did the female victims. These self-reports may be accurate and reflective of actual differences in degree of abuse, but the self-reports also may reflect a male tendency to minimize injury and emotional impact. Mouton et al. (2001) reported men in a focus group setting expressing hurt feelings about verbal abuse, suggesting that such feelings may be harbored, but not expressed under normal circumstances. In our study we found widowers minimizing their efforts and burdens as caregivers for ill wives (Moore & Stratton, 2002). Kaye (1997) found similar tendencies among male caregivers. When grandfathers had conflict with younger generations of their family, they tended to minimize the conflict and avoided dealing with the problems (Boxer, Cook, & Cohler, 1986). Boxer et al. suggest that the older men minimize conflict so as not to alienate the ones who will be giving care. An interesting example of masculine minimizing involved a 70-year-old father not able or willing to express responsibility for his earlier abusive behavior and then minimizing the recent gestures he had made during family therapy to reconcile with his son (Mauldin & Anderson, 1998).

Not seeking help. Widowed men "are reported to be among the most recalcitrant and difficult of people to assist" (Campbell & Silverman, 1996, p. 20). Boxer et al. (1986) note that men have what amounts to a "ban on expressiveness" (p. 96) that would curtail any inclination to tell someone what they feel. Men suffering from depression are also reluctant to seek help (McIntosh, Pearson, & Lebowitz, 1997). Kosberg (1998) found men are more likely to self-medicate with alcohol and are more likely to self-abuse, including suicide. Pritchard (2001) found men expressing a sense of duty and loyalty to their children, which resulted in failing to report mistreatment.

Not trying to repair fractured relationships. Again, the tendency to avoid expressiveness (Boxer, Cook, & Cohler, 1986) might keep men from attempting to repair relationships. Edelman (2006) identifies four types of fathers, as she examines men's ways of relating to their young daughters following the death of their wives, These types grow out of the men's personalities and coping styles and would, therefore, continue in parent-adult child relationships. The "Heroic" type is a consistent support in his children's lives, managing his own grief and allowing them to express theirs. The other three types, however, are rooted in some dysfunction and would lend themselves to relationship fractures. The "I'm OK, You're OK" father does not allow for mourning–his own or his child's. Edelman describes this response to the father's loss as "silence, avoidance, and remarriage." The "Helpless" type of father cannot cope with his wife's death and expects the daughter to take care of him. The "Distant" type is usually distant before the wife's death and responds to her death by becoming even more distant from his children. Edelman's categories are a reminder that ways of grieving and adjusting are highly individual and will impact relationships differentially. Consistent across the less-functional types, however, is the tendency not to face a sad reality and therefore not move forward from it in a positive way. If the basic loss cannot be faced, then the resulting relationship fractures cannot be understood and appropriately responded to.

Difficult personalities. "Difficult" personalities were evidenced in several of the interviews, attitudes that carried beyond father-child relationships to a general way of viewing and dealing with life. However, intensity seemed to gather at the point of the father-child relationship, and leads us to wonder if these generally negative fathers are externalizing a sense of failure about their own parenting. This, in turn, may result in blaming a child for having grown up irresponsible or for making poor choices, and accusing the wife (now deceased) of having coddled the child. Nydegger and Mitteness (1991) found fathers to be more critical of their sons, as did we in some notable cases of alienation. They also found, as did we, that relationships could differ greatly from child to child. Some of our men were alienated from only one child, thus keeping at least some possibilities of emotional, social and material support from their other adult children. Is this a strategy to assure future assistance–to keep good relations with at least one child?

Personalities/Characteristics of the Adult Children

"It takes two to tango," as the old saying goes. Fulmer et al. (2005) found the personality of both the neglectful child and the neglected elder to be characterized by statistically significant factors in already determined neglect cases, and that a "mutual influence" contributed to elder neglect. Anetzberger (1987) described types of abusive adult children. The hostile child has had a long-term poor relationship with the parent and is angry and aggressive. The authoritarian child is rigid, punitive, and domineering. The dependent child is not so easily described, but is always financially dependent on the parent and is generally "pathetic" and "immature." There is more chance of neglect when adult children have serious problems of their own, such as substance abuse, marital discord, or marital breakup (Greenberg & Becker, 1988). Tomita (1990), basing her work on Sykes and Matza (1957), describes how caregivers avoid guilt or shame for their abusive or neglectful behaviors by using strategies (techniques of neutralization) to rationalize or justify their mistreatment of elders.

We obviously have an interest in the personalities of the adult children who were part of fractured relationships in our study. However, we typically heard only the father's description of the child and his version of the relationship problems. It did seem that some of the children were "difficult." Russell's daughter was managing to manipulate him constantly into giving her money. George claimed his one son even might not make time to have lunch with him, even if he went to his son's town.

We did speak with Walter's daughter; she seemed sad and sullen. She said she regretted that her father had not broken away from his harsh family of origin who poorly related to each other. She felt that she had taken on many of her father's traits and that her own life quality was diminished as a result. Walter lived out his life with a new wife whose bubbly personality helped her perceive everything in a positive light. But if she had predeceased Walter, it is highly unlikely that Walter's children would have wanted to take care of him or include him in their lives. Walter and his children are an example of family context and early life experiences that can lead to the risk of neglect.

In such families, neglectful behavior may have been modeled for the children by their parent; the children may have been the direct victims of such treatment. They could be retaliating for treatment received from the father in childhood or retaliating for treatment suffered by the mother (Tatara, 1993). Neglect could also reflect other resentments of various sorts. On the other hand, Karl's son and Curly's son gave caring attention to their harsh fathers, so the interplay of personality dynamics will be an important factor in determining how care vs. neglect possibilities actually work out.

Contact and Quality in the Father-Child Relationship

In general. Suitor, Pillemer, Keeton, and Robison (1995) and Nydegger and Mitteness (1991) found that relationship quality between an older parent and adult child improves with the child's age. Fingerman (2001) explains intimacy in a healthy parent/adult child relationship as a "distant closeness." Because of their respect for each other as adult individuals, they recognize each other's strengths and weaknesses. Closeness involves allowing each other to have some privacy and trusting each to manage his or her own life. This kind of closeness allows for adjustments acceptable to both, as the elderly parent begins to need more care. Often, however, relationships carry baggage from the past that does not fully allow for such mature intimacy.

Common wisdom holds that adult children have closer relationships with their mothers than with their fathers. Research seems to bear that out (Hoffman, McManus, & Brackbill, 1987; Troll & Fingerman, as cited in Fingerman, 2001). Primary to this is the role of the mother as "kinkeeper" of the family, the one who maintains contact and brings family members together (Hagestad, 1986). Lawton, Silverstein, and Bengtson (1994) found that affection between fathers and adult children did not necessarily lead to more contact, as was the case with mothers. Fathers tended to be more likely to accept an invitation rather than to initiate an arrangement for visits. Death of the mother affects the amount of contact; as if fathers and children have trouble managing to get together without the mother, the kinkeeper, to arrange it (Aquilino, 1994). Nakonezny, Rodgers, and Nussbaum (2003) noted this same pattern when families were disrupted by divorce.

Specifically after widowhood. Stereotypes of men having an easier time with bereavement–just wanting a housekeeper, just wanting sex, quickly replacing a wife–may lead friends and family to underestimate the depth of grieving and the needs of the widowed man (Campbell & Silverman, 1996). Van den Hoonaard (2001) describes widowed women and their children as trying to establish "a balance between privacy and support" in their daily interactions (p. 45). This is in contrast to the research findings on widowed men and their children, whose relationship issues after death of the wife/mother often center on lack of contact, lower quality of relationship, and sometimes estrangement (Aquilino, 1994).

Aquilino (1994) found mothers and daughters have a relationship of reciprocal helpfulness, which is not affected by divorce or death of the father. However, a daughter loses that help exchange when her mother dies; her widowed father cannot provide the same level of reciprocity, and so their relationship weakens, while the father-son relationship seems to remain the same. Nydegger and Mitteness (1991) describe father-son relationships as more complex and more criticism-prone, yet based on shared activities and perspectives. Suitor et al. (1995) find that fathers are closer to their daughters than to their sons. Our study found some daughters giving their widowed fathers a great deal of help and that brought complications to their relationship, especially when the father repartnered. These complications will be considered further in the context of remarriage later in this article.

In contrast to divorce, widowhood seems to strengthen a child's sense of obligation to support the surviving parent (Aquilino, 1994). Also, widowed fathers continued to contribute financially to adult children, suggesting what might be a man's way of showing that he cares (Aquilino,

1994; Hoffman, McManus, & Brackbill, 1987). Men in our study who had made careful plans about their finances tended to have good relationships with their children. Some of the men we interviewed had decided not to remarry because of financial complexities. Some of the remarried men had made prenuptial agreements to keep finances clear. The children may have been more at ease when they knew that Dad had provided for himself and that inheritance matters were settled.

Conflict in the Father-Child Relationship

Abusive caregiving children can express ambivalence in the caregiving role (Anetzberger, 1987). The adult child seems to want to give care but can find the burdens great, especially in terms of lack of independence and free time and the failure of other family members to give enough assistance. Steinman (as cited in Cicirelli, 1986) describes three types of conflict in later life when adult children are called upon to assist an elder parent: continuing conflict, reactivated conflict, and new conflict. Brody (1985) refers to "incompletely resolved crises [being] reprised" (p. 23), and indicates that children report conflicts with parents related to the parent's health and things the child thought the parent should do, the parent's temperament, and his or her tendency to criticize or make demands. Cicirelli reports that adult children expected more conflict with mothers than with fathers, should the elder parent come to live with them. However, Suitor, Pillemer, Keeton, and Robison. (1995), in a review of the literature, concluded that there is greater conflict in the father-son relationship than in any other dyad.

Boxer, Cook, and Cohler (1986) found grandfathers to idealize their relationships and to perceive less conflict with sons and grandsons than the younger generations perceived. Nydegger and Mitteness (1991) similarly found fathers perceiving less conflict than did their adult sons and daughters. A mismatch of perceptions could lead an older man to underestimate the alienation felt by his potential caregivers, the younger generations of his family.

In our study we found evidence that early harsh or emotionally distant fathering was at the origin of some parent-adult child conflict. The vehemence of George's negativity about one son and his wife's "coddling" role, and his fight-the-world attitude about some other matters led us to think he might have been harsh in his parenting. Yussef had a very stern look and demeanor, although he was a very willing participant in the study. He expressed terse disapproval of one son who he felt was not responsible and was coddled by the mother all his life. He expressed high approval of the other son, who apparently consulted him when making important decisions. George also approved of one son and disapproved of the other, but his opinion of each was much more extreme. He spoke of the approved son as always being there for him, even though they lived several hundred miles apart. He then went on to describe incidents in which he had become very verbally forceful with his irresponsible son. It appeared to the interviewer that they had cut off all contact after the wife/mother's sudden death. Walter presented a particularly dramatic picture of harsh and distant parenting. He never referred to his children by name, but called them "the boy" and "the girl." His daughter, referred to earlier, expressed much bitterness toward him, but seemed fond of his second wife. Alvin and his son's wife did not get along. He told the interviewer the woman was "ugly" and could not tolerate her mother-in-law's attractiveness. He described decades with almost no contact and had directly accused the son of participating in the withdrawal to please his wife. Malcolm also complained of not getting along with a daughter-in-law, but to a lesser degree. Distance and travel costs were convenient reasons for not visiting each other.

These fathers were very different from each other in terms of religious backgrounds, occupations and income levels, and interests in life. However, they had personalities that came through as critical and controlling, as they related stories in the interviews. In situations of very harsh parenting, conflict and withdrawal were not inevitable. In the two cases of harsh parenting reported by adult children, the children had risen to an admirable level of caring for the elder father in spite of their harsh upbringing. Karl's son is a pastor and gave loving care in spite of Karl's earlier domineering behavior toward the son and mother. Curly's son seemed a bit cowered by his father's lifelong control, but took steps to protect his mother in her failing old age and then was attentive to his father in his failing old age.

CONTEXTS FOR POTENTIAL NEGLECT

Pagelow (1988) and Pillemer and Finkelhor (1988) found that the elderly are most likely to be abused by those with whom they live. Older males are more likely to live with another person and, thus, are at risk for abuse. Fulmer et al. (2005) found neglected elders living with fewer people in the household; those who live alone are more likely to be neglected. When the older father and adult child are living separately, as they were in our study, and perhaps with infrequent contact, the situation could likely result in neglect. Beyond these general circumstances, there are configurations of family disruption that can increase the risk of neglect. We will consider remarriage, circumstances with stepchildren, and divorce.

Remarriage

Older widowers are more likely than widows to be interested in remarrying and to actually re-marry. Strobe and Schut (as cited in Riches & Dawson, 2000) describe widowers as having a strategy of "restoration," that is, repairing disrupted routines, which often means restoring the lost marital situation with a new partner. Two studies of widowers found that older (over age 80), less healthy men gave up on the idea of remarriage and more of them stated that their deceased wife could never be replaced, but younger and healthier widowers were interested in a new partner to deal with their loneliness (Davidson, 2001; Moore & Stratton, 2002). Our study noted respondents describing evenings alone at home as particularly difficult. Davidson concluded that widows want a companion to go out with in a couples-oriented society, while widowers want a companion to come home to.

Davidson (2001) also describes widowed women as less interested in remarriage because they see marriage as a constant exercise in attending to the wants and needs of the husband. Most of the women interviewed in Davidson's study were enjoying their freedom and did not want to take on another caring duty of that magnitude. This raises the possibility that a widowed woman could remarry but then discover her dislike of returning to a caregiving role. A new wife may not have the feelings of devotion and obligation for care that often develop in a long-term marriage. We interviewed one man who had suffered a major stroke a month after his remarriage. At the time of the interview it did not appear there was abuse or neglect occurring, but his previously-widowed wife expressed great disappointment that she was now so limited by this invalid man. When remarried women are disillusioned with their second marriages, discord and the possibility of mistreatment increase (Ron & Lowenstein, 1999).

As noted earlier, children can feel alienated from the father by his quick remarriage, which represents a replacement of their irreplaceable mother (Edelman, 2006; Lester & Lester, 1980; Lund, Caserta, & Dimond, 1993; Moore & Stratton, 2002; Riches & Dawson, 2000). Even if they do not feel alienated, the children may not be sure of their caregiving responsibility in light of the new marriage situation. Or, other issues—such as finances and family alliances—can surface. In our study, Sy had been remarried for more than 20 years, but came to a point at which his children convinced him to leave his wife over a conflicted financial situation involving the adult children of the two spouses. His children had no regard for his emotional attachment to his wife, and manipulated him, while he was ill and dependent, into choosing to leave her and go to their home state with them. This seems clearly to be a case of emotional mistreatment.

We also encountered two instances of very recent upsets about remarriage. Earl's daughter could not accept his remarriage even though she had encouraged him to date; Stuart's son could not accept that a new wife lived in the home previously shared by his father and mother. Both fathers were hoping the child would eventually accept the new marriage but were not actively trying to repair the relationship. Stuart said his wife was trying to be a good grandmother to the son's children, and he hoped that the children's acceptance of her would eventually bring the son's approval. Earl hoped his daughter would understand he needed a new partner.

With 11 children, Cordell faced a variety of responses to his personality and his behavior. He was a very self-assured man and seemed to come off as arrogant and controlling to some of his children. One daughter in particular seemed dismayed at his rapid repartnering. She asked him, "Do you ever think of Mom?" Since an adult child cannot replace a parent, a father's repartnering can seem like a callous replacement of a beloved parent.

Our study found that nearly every man had found a "current woman" who fulfilled roles of the departed wife (Moore & Stratton, 2002; Moore & Stratton, 2004). The "current woman" could be a new wife, a companion, a neighbor, a friend, a daughter or daughter-in-law or granddaughter. This offers another possible explanation for father-daughter conflict: a lack of agreement on their reconfigured gender relationship. Particularly in the case of a daughter who feels she has taken care of her widowed father, the father's repartnering can be perceived as a betrayal. A daughter may first identify with a beloved woman–the mother–who can be quickly replaced and second identify with a caring woman–herself–who is seen not as important as a new partner. A son also can feel that his father has replaced someone (his mother) who is irreplaceable to him.

Stepchildren and Alienation

Clawson and Ganong (2002) interviewed older stepparents and adult stepchildren and found them agreeing (mostly hypothetically) that stepchildren are not obligated to assist. Nevertheless, the children gave several positive reasons that they would be inclined to help, including *the* quality of their relationship with the stepparent, if the stepparent reared them, if the stepparent had been a good spouse to their parent, and if the stepparent had helped them in adulthood. Eggebeen (1992) found a strong negative relationship between stepchild status and actually giving support to an elder stepparent, but speculates that those stepchildren who had been reared for years by the stepparent would have increased motivation to give care.

Our study had three cases of fractured step-relationships: Robert did not accept his wife's out-of-wedlock son as family. Even though the son tried to be caring and helpful, a willing source of support was cut off. Leroy felt stressed his wife's son did not give him more attention, as he felt he had put a lot of effort into helping to raise him. The son invited him to a family dinner about once a month, but always seemed to be too busy to sit and talk with him. Bert said he had never gotten along with his wife's daughter who was 13 when they married; they had no contact after his wife died.

Divorce

Although our study did not involve men who had ended their marriages through divorce, our findings about men's difficulties in maintaining relationships with adult children raise concerns for growing numbers of men who have lost contact and perhaps filial affection because of divorce. Studies utilizing the 1988 National Survey of Families and Households conclude that divorce negatively impacts father-adult child relationships in a number of ways. Aquilino (1994) found that father-child relationships deteriorated more than did mother-child relationships. Also, parental divorce weakens a child's sense of obligation to support parents, while widowhood seems to strengthen it. Cooney and Uhlenberg (1990) found that "divorce has pronounced negative effects on men's contacts with their adult offspring and on their perceptions of adult children as potential sources of support in times of need" (p. 85). Altfeld (1995) concluded that family disruption profoundly affects intergenerational contact, quality of relationships, and availability of care for frail elderly fathers. Eggebeen (1992) refers to this lack of support as "disquieting" in light of the growing number of divorced elders.

Webster and Herzog (1995) found that children reported lower quality relationships with their parents when they had memories of family problems. Divorce lowered the quality even more. Children of divorce were much less likely to have positive relationships with their fathers. Divorce also led to significantly reduced communication between parents and their children, with the effects more pronounced for fathers. Lawton, Silverstein, and Bengtson (1994) likewise noted that divorce diminishes both affection and frequency of contact between fathers and their adult children.

The effects of older-age parental divorces may be felt acutely by children and may dramatically affect behaviors, especially if older divorced parents need assistance while children are still processing their own emotional transition in the divorce situation (Nakonezny, Rodgers, & Nussbaum, 2003). A buffering effect provided by the long term stability of the parent-child bond did seem to help stabilize relationships at the time of divorce. However, that effect seemed to work for mother-child relationships much more than for father-child relationships. Nakonezny et al. attribute this difference to the mothers being more "giving" as traditional kinkeepers. Mothers have the motivation and the skills to maintain this central role in their lives in spite of divorce, whereas divorcing fathers typically withdraw or are isolated.

These research findings illuminate patterns of relationship stress and degrees of fracture that typically result in adult children feeling less connected with and responsible for their divorced fathers. While we did not study fathers of divorce, we feel this growing population of men may face old age and possible dependency with little in the way of family support systems to call upon.

THEORTETICAL PERSPECTIVES
ON THE POTENTIAL FOR NEGLECT

Thus far we have examined factors and dynamics that seem to create a high risk for neglect. Yet, there are many individuals and families caring for elders even when early relationships or events along the way have not been positive. There must be forces working against the negativity in many families. There is usually a combination of affection and sense of duty in caregiving situations, so we will look at theories relating to obligation and attachment for some insights. These theories also help us to understand what dynamics can lead to neglect.

Obligation. Obligation is a theme of central importance to the elder parent-adult child relationship. It was a matter of great pride to our respondent Louis that his children and grandchildren did not visit him out of a sense of duty, but instead really enjoyed spending time with him.

Our respondent Sy felt his own children were properly attentive but bitterly judged his wife's sons as minimally performing their filial obligations. In making this comparison known to his children through the years, he unwittingly created what became a battle of accusations between the two sets of adult children and a bitter struggle over finances, which resulted in the permanent separation of the elderly and ailing spouses.

Altfeld (1995) finds women have a greater sense of filial duty. Lawton et al. (1994) describe the father-child relationship as more instrumental or obligatory than affectionate. Whitbeck, Simons, and Conger (1991) found a small positive correlation (statistically significant for sons, not significant for daughters) between quality of current relationship and caregiving. Positive early relationships contributed to positive current relationships, which increased the motivation for caregiving. The caregiving experience adds stress to the adult child's life (Brody, 1985), which can in itself cause stress in the relationship and affect motivation. Whitbeck et al. also found some children caring for a parent in spite of rating the current relationship quality as low. A sense of obligation that developed through the years apparently prevailed. Particularly in situations where early relationships were positive, the obligation to provide care buffers the negative aspects of caregiving.

Caregiving out of a sense of obligation does not guarantee good care. Physical care can be delivered in a minimal or perfunctory way which can still convey degrees of neglect. Perfunctory visits can leave an elderly person feeling unvalued and emotionally neglected. Our respondent Leroy, mentioned earlier, felt neglected by his stepson in spite of regular contact.

Attachment. Attachment is a lifelong continuation of the child's emotional bond with the parent. In the parent's old age the child exhibits attachment behaviors such as living close to the parent and keeping in frequent contact (Cicirelli, 1986). As the parent's dependency increases, the child will exhibit more attachment behaviors. These behaviors increase the feelings of attachment and the commitment to provide assistance in the future. A sense of filial obligation also plays a role. However, it is the strong feelings of attachment that help a caregiver deal with negative feelings, such as frustration and resentment, that naturally develop as the helping burden increases. We saw the attachment penomenon at a very high level with two of our centenarian widowers. Ned was adored and celebrated by his children and their spouses. Eldon had a parade of family members stopping in at the little home he insisted on staying in alone; there were frustrations with his stubbornness, but familial attachment grew to meet his needs under his terms.

Social exchange. Social exchange refers to social interaction being based on actions that are expected to bring returns (Blau, 1964). In essence, people do what they do with an expectation of some sort of benefit. Expectations in a relationship change as years pass and circumstances change. Thomas (1994) describes the process of managing these changes as "maintaining a dynamic balance" (p. 203). This seemed to be the case in the families of most of our respondents. Al's children were not available to him, but Al created a strong reciprocity with his granddaughter that helped get his needs met. He gave her family the money to put an addition on their house; she took him to all his appointments and shopping. Fathers gave advice, money, and/or companionship to their families; in return, families provided for the man's current needs (Moore & Stratton, 2002). Some families, however, do not maintain a balance. Sy, mentioned earlier, felt he and his wife had "invested" equally in both sets of adult children, but received much more contact and attention in return from his children. He was bitter about his stepchildren's "negligence," as they had not lived up to his standard of reciprocity.

Benefits can be intangible, such as feeling that one is doing one's duty or feeling appreciated as a good son or daughter. Generally when behaviors do not bring expected benefits, the lack of adequate rewards can end or change the relationship (Gelles, 1983). It is not easy to end a family relationship, so stress is played out within the relationship. Brody (1985) views increasing parental dependency as disrupting the family homeostasis. A parent who is not appreciative enough in the opinion of the caregiver, or whose care is causing stress far beyond any balancing rewards to the caregiver, may find the caregiver becoming neglectful. Also, negative behaviors can result in positive benefits, such as a feeling of power and self-righteousness when controlling someone else. Misappropriating a parent's money results in ample and tangible rewards. If there is no social control such as legal action or social disapproval on the child who is doing it, the behavior will continue (Gelles). The isolation of an elder reduces the possibility of social controls on the behavior of whoever has caregiving responsibility and, as a result, makes abuse or neglect more likely.

CONCLUSIONS

As we have explored the potential for neglect of elderly men, a complex picture emerges. Personal factors of both parties and their relationship dynamics are interwoven with the family's life events and abstract motivations such as attachment, sense of duty, and reciprocity. Langer's (1990) study of grandparents and grandchildren describes the configuration of factors that determine the extent of support as "history of assistance, individual characteristics, and the emotional ties shared by the pair" (p. 109).

Our own study of widowed men allowed us to look more closely at the men's perspectives on family relationships. From that study, we note several tendencies that would seem to increase the risk of neglect. Men tend not to be active kinkeepers; their relationships with family often diminish after the death of their spouses. Personality and personal style affect men's relationships with their children in ways that can contribute to conflict and therefore increase the potential for withdrawal and ultimately neglect. The men in our study were not attempting to repair fractured relationships. Some of them hoped the relationships would improve, and some did not seem to care if relationships improved. But none took steps to improve them.

We see a pattern of "masculine minimizing" that is broader than we had originally recognized. Men tend to minimize their feelings and their problems and are therefore not likely to seek help, thus increasing the risk for victimization. Additionally, by minimizing their own emotions, they may not be aware of how their behaviors (for example, expressions of anger) have been perceived by their child, or how their child has been affected. The literature shows older men tending to minimize the conflict in their family relationships, so they may not be aware of the degree of anger or alienation felt by an adult child.

We see affection and sense of duty as strong motivating factors for adult children who find themselves needing to care for an elder parent. However, in the case of fractured relationships, that motivation may be extinguished or never called upon. The withdrawal of children and their fathers from each other as a response to conflict is a possible precursor to neglect. Withdrawal could lead to adult children not being aware of the father's current needs, even if they would be willing to help. Also, in the absence of substantial interaction, family relationships may grow weaker even when there is no conflict. Little or no contact would probably continue even when the father's needs increase.

Remarriage can bring significant benefits to a widower's life, but also can introduce conflict that increases the risk of abuse and neglect. Finally, while we did not interview divorced men, we feel that, from our review of the literature, divorce often lowers frequency of contact and the quality of father-child relationships, thereby increasing the possible risk that the children will not come to their father's aid in his old age.

SUGGESTIONS FOR FURTHER STUDY

The "masculine minimizing" tendency can be pervasive and complex, as we have just described above, and should lead researchers to be skeptical of self-reports by older men. Researchers should design methodologies that will reveal and explore the minimizing tendency.

There is a need to determine if older men who tend to be less critical and more accepting in old age have changed because they are not so concerned about traditional masculinity any longer or because it is a strategy to keep a potential caregiver in a positive relationship. Further, research can reveal whether there is a strategy for long-term reciprocity that guides aging parents–fathers and mothers–in their relationships with children.

The situation of divorce and father-child relationships is worthy of further study (Cooney & Uhlenberg, 1990). It may be possible to improve family support systems for some men, but also service providers will be called upon to create supportive programming to stand in place of family relationships when they realistically are not available to some men. In both cases the goal would be to minimize the possible self-neglect, neglect and abandonment situations that could result.

REFERENCES

Altfeld, S. J. (1995). *Caring for elderly fathers: The impact of family disruption.* Unpublished doctoral dissertation, University of Illinois at Chicago.

Anetzberger, G. J. (1987). *The etiology of elder abuse by adult offspring.* Springfield, IL: Charles C Thomas.

Aquilino, W. S. (1994). Later life parental divorce and widowhood: Impact on young adults' assessment of parent-child relations. *Journal of Marriage and the Family, 56*(4), 908-922.

Blau, P. M. (1964). *Exchange and power in social life.* New York: John Wiley & Sons.

Boxer, A. M., Cook, J. A. & Cohler, B. J. (1986). Grandfathers, fathers, and sons: Inter-generational relations among men. In K. A. Pillemer & R. S. Wolf (Eds.), *Elder abuse: Conflict in the family* (pp. 93-121). Dover, MA: Auburn House.

Brody, E. M. (1985). Parent care as a normative family stress. *The Gerontologist, 25,* 19-29.

Butler, R. N. (1969). Age-ism: Another form of bigotry. *The Gerontologist, 9,* 243-246.

Campbell, S. & Silverman, P. R. (1996). *Widower: When men are left alone.* Amityville, NY: Baywood.

Circirelli, V. G. (1986). The helping relationship and family neglect in later life. In K. A. Pillemer & R. S. Wolf (Eds.). *Elder abuse: Conflict in the family* (pp. 49-66). Dover, MA: Auburn House.

Clawson, J. & Ganong, L. (2002). Adult stepchildren's obligations to older stepparents. *Journal of Family Nursing, 8*(1), 50-72.

Cooney, T. & Uhlenberg, P. (1990). The role of divorce in men's relations with their adult children after mid-life. *Journal of Marriage and the Family, 52*(3), 677-688.

Davidson, K. (2001). Late life widowhood, selfishness and new partnership choices: A gendered perspective. *Aging & Society, 21*, 297-317.

Edelman, H. (2006). *Motherless daughters: The legacy of loss* (2nd ed). Cambridge, MA: Da Capo Press.

Eggebeen, D. J. (1992). Family structure and intergenerational exchanges. *Research on Aging, 14*(4), 427-447.

Fingerman, K. L. (2001). A distant closeness: Intimacy between parents and their children in later life. *Generations, 25*(2), 26-33.

Fulmer, T., Paveza, G., VandeWeerd, C., Fairchild, S., Guadagno, L., Bolton-Blatt, M., & Norman, R. (2005). Dyadic vulnerability and risk profiling for elder neglect. *The Gerontologist, 45*(4), 525-534.

Gelles, R. J. (1983). An exchange/social control theory. In D. Finkelhor, R. J. Gelles, G. T. Hataling, & M. A. Straus (Eds.), *The dark side of families: Current family violence research* (pp. 151-165).

Glasser, B. C. & Strauss, A. L. (1967). *The discovering of grounded theory: Strategies for qualitative research.* New York: Aldine de Gruyter.

Greenberg, J. S. (1991). Problems in the lives of adult children: Their impact on aging parents. *Journal of Gerontological Social Work, 16*, 149-161.

Greenberg, J. S. & Becker, M. (1988). Aging parents as family resources. *The Gerontologist, 28*(6), 786-791.

Hagestad, G. O. (1986, Winter). The aging society as a context for family life. *Daedaelus, 115*(1), 119-140.

Hoffman, L. W., McManus, K. A., & Brackbill, Y. (1987). The value of children to young and elderly parents. *International Journal of Aging and Human Development, 25*(4), 309-322.

Hwalek, M., Goodrich, C. S., & Quinn, K. (1996). In L. A. Baumhover & S. C. Beall (Eds.). *Abuse, neglect, and exploitation of older persons: Strategies for assessment & intervention* (pp. 31-49). Baltimore: Health Professions Press.

Kaye, L. (1997). Informal caregiving by older men. In J. I. Kosberg & L. W. Kaye (Eds.). *Elderly men: Special problems and professional challenges* (pp. 231-249). New York: Springer Publishing.

Kosberg, J. I. (1998). The abuse of elderly men. *Journal of Elder Abuse & Neglect, 9*(3), 69-88.

Kosberg, J. I. & Nahmiash, D. (1996). Characteristics of victims and perpetrators and milieus of abuse and neglect. In L. A. Baumhover & S. C. Beall (Eds.), *Abuse, neglect, and exploitation of older persons: Strategies for assessment and intervention* (pp. 31-49). Baltimore: Health Professions Press.

Langer, N. (1990). Grandparents and adult grandchildren: What do they do for one another? *International Journal of Aging and Human Development, 31*(2), 101-110.

Lawton. L., Silverstein, M., & Bengtson, V. (1994). Affection, social contact, and geographic distance between adult children and their parents. *Journal of Marriage and the Family, 56*(1), 57-68.

Lester, A. D. & Lester, J. L. (1980). *Understand aging parents.* Philadelphia, PA: The Westminster Press.

Lund, D. A., Caserta, M. S., & Dimond, M. F. (1993). Spousal bereavement in later life. In M. S. Stroebe, W. Stroebe, & R. O. Hansson (Eds.), *Handbook of bereavement* (pp. 240-254). New York: Cambridge University Press.

Mauldin, G. R. & Anderson, W. T. (1998). Forgiveness as an intervention in contextual family therapy: Two case examples. *TCA Journal, 26*(2), 123-132.

McIntosh, J. L., Pearson, J. L., & Lebowitz, B. D. (1997). Mental disorders of elderly men. In J. I. Kosberg & L. W. Kaye (Eds.), *Elderly men: Special problems and professional challenges* (pp. 193-215). New York: Springer Publishing.

Moore, A. J. & Stratton, D. C. (2002). *Resilient widowers: Older men speak for themselves.* New York: Springer Publishing.

Moore, A. J. & Stratton, D. C. (2004). The current woman in an older widower's life. In G. Fennell & K. Davidson (Eds.), *Intimacy in later life* (pp. 121-142). New Brunswick, NJ: Transaction.

Mouton, C. P., Talamantes, M., Parker, R. W., Espino, D. V., & Miles, T. P. (2001). Abuse and neglect in older men. *Clinical Gerontologist, 24*(3/4), 15-26.

Nakonezny, P. A., Rodgers, J. L., & Nussbaum, J. F. (2003). The effect of later life parental divorce on adult-child/older-parent solidarity: A test of the buffering hypothesis. *Journal of applied Social Psychology, 33*(6), 1153-1178.

National Center on Elder Abuse at the American Public Human Services Association in Collaboration with Westat, Inc. (1998). *The national elder abuse incidence study: Final report.* Washington, DC: National Aging Information Center.

Nydegger, C. N. & Mitteness, L. S. (1991). Father and their adult sons and daughters. *Marriage and the Family Review, 16*, 245-256.

Pagelow, M. D. (1988). Abuse of the elderly in the home. In A. L. Horton & J. A. Williamson (Eds.), *Abuse and religion: When praying isn't enough* (pp. 29-38). Lexington, MA: Lexington Books.

Pillemer, K. & Finkelhor, D. (1988). The prevalence of elder abuse: A random sample survey. *The Gerontologist, 28*(1), 51-57.

Pillemer, K. A. & Wolf, R. S. (Eds.) (1986). *Elder abuse: Conflict in the family.* Dover, MA: Auburn House.

Pillemer, K. & Finkelhor, D. (1989). Causes of elder abuse: Caregiver stress versus problem relatives. *American Journal of Orthopsychiatry, 29*(2), 179-187.

Pritchard, J. (2001). *Male victims of elder abuse.* London: Jessica Kingsley.

Riches, G. & Dawson, P. (2000). Daughters' dilemmas: Grief resolution in girls whose widowed father remarry early. *Journal of Family Therapy, 22*(4), 360-374.

Ron, P. & Lowenstein, A. (1999). Loneliness and unmet needs of intimacy and sexuality: Their effect on the phenomenon of spousal abuse in second marriages of the widowed elder. *Journal of Divorce & Remarriage, 31*(3/4),

Steinmetz, S. K. (1977-78). The battered husband syndrome. *Victimology, 2*(3/4), 499-509.

Suitor, J. J., Pillemer, K., Keeton, S., & Robison, J. (1995). Aged parents and aging children: Determinants of relationship quality. In R. Blieszner & V. H. Bedford (Eds.). *Handbook of aging and the family,* (pp. 221-242). Westport, CT: Greenwood Press.

Sykes, G. & Matza, D. (1957). Techniques of neutralization. A theory of delinquency. *American Sociological Review, 22,* 664-670.

Tatara, T. (1993). Understanding the nature and scope of domestic elder abuse with the use of state aggregate data: Summaries of the key findings of a national survey of state APS and aging agencies. *Journal of Elder Abuse & Neglect, 5*(4), 35-59.

Thomas, J. L. (1994). Older men as fathers and grandfathers. In E. H. Thompson Jr. (Ed.) *Older men's lives* (pp. 197-217). Thousand Oaks, CA: Sage Publications.

Tomita, S. K. (1990). The denial of elder mistreatment by victims and abusers: The application of neutralization theory. *Violence and Victims, 5*(3), 171-184.

Van den Hoonaard, D. K. (2001). *The widowed self: The older woman's journey through widowhood.* Waterloo, ON: Wilfrid Laurier University Press.

Webster, P. S. & Herzog, A. R. (1995). Effects of parental divorce and memories of family problems on relationships between adult children and their parents. *Journals of Gerontology, 50B*(1), S 524-534.

Whitbeck. L. B., Simons, R. L., & Conger, R. D. (1991). The effects of early family relationships on contemporary relationships and assistance patterns between adult children and their parents. *Journals of Gerontology, 46B*(6), S330-337.

Whittaker, T. (1996). Violence, gender and elder abuse. In B. Fawcett, B. Featherstone, J. Hearn, & C. Toft (Eds.), *Violence & gender relations: Theories and interventions* (pp. 147-160). London: Sage Publications.

Wolf, R. S. (1996). Understanding elder abuse and neglect. *Aging, 367,* 4-13.

doi:10.1300/J084v19n01_06

Notes on Newspaper Accounts
of Male Elder Abuse

R. L. McNeely, PhD, JD
Philip W. Cook, BS

SUMMARY. Law enforcement press releases and other print-media miscellany detailing accounts of male elder abuse involving insurance fraud, false allegations by perpetrators, and abuse inflicted by caregivers, spawned interest in a more systematic review. That review was accomplished principally by accessing two search engines, with news articles from 1986 to the present. A review of these media accounts transformed the initial "insurance fraud" category into a broader one classified as "economic exploitation." That same review also resulted in three distinctive categories of caregiver abuse. This article provides abbreviated case accounts within each category, and concludes with brief notes on several themes derived from the reported accounts. doi:10.1300/ J084v19n01_07 *[Article copies available for a fee from The Haworth Document Delivery Service: 1-800-HAWORTH. E-mail address: <docdelivery@ haworthpress.com> Website: <http://www.HaworthPress.com> © 2007 by The Haworth Press, Inc. All rights reserved.]*

R. L. McNeely is a practicing attorney and Professor of Social Welfare at the University of Wisconsin-Milwaukee, Bader School of Social Welfare, Milwaukee, WI 53216 (E-mail: rlmatty@ticon.net). Philip W. Cook is an author, journalist, and President of Arrowdot Productions, Inc., P.O. Box 951, Tualatin, OR 97062 (E-mail: Philip. cook@comcast.net).

[Haworth co-indexing entry note]: "Notes on Newspaper Accounts of Male Elder Abuse." McNeely, R. L., and Philip W. Cook. Co-published simultaneously in *Journal of Elder Abuse & Neglect*™ (The Haworth Maltreatment & Trauma Press®, an imprint of The Haworth Press, Inc.) Vol. 19, No. 1/2, 2007, pp. 99-108; and: *Abuse of Older Men* (ed: Jordan I. Kosberg) The Haworth Maltreatment & Trauma Press®, an imprint of The Haworth Press, Inc., 2007, pp. 99-108. Single or multiple copies of this article are available for a fee from The Haworth Document Delivery Service [1-800-HAWORTH, 9:00 a.m. - 5:00 p.m. (EST). E-mail address: docdelivery@haworthpress.com].

Available online at http://jean.haworthpress.com
© 2007 by The Haworth Press, Inc. All rights reserved.
doi:10.1300/J084v19n01_07

KEYWORDS. Aging, domestic violence, caregiver abuse, elder abuse, economic exploitation, male elder abuse, male domestic violence victims

INTRODUCTION

A review of recent newspaper accounts detailing the abuse of elderly men yielded five categories of violence. That review was accomplished principally by accessing two search engines, *ProQuest Newspapers* and *Newpaper Archive.com*. *ProQuests* surveys 550 US and international news sources including more than 150 major newspapers, detailing news articles from 1986 to the present. *Newspaper Archive.com* surveys more than 2500 newspaper titles ranging as far back in time as 1759. A review of media accounts appearing since 1986 transformed the initial "insurance fraud" category into a broader category classified as "economic exploitation." That same review also resulted in three distinctive categories of caregiver abuse.

The five categories of abuse include cases involving: (a) economic abuse; (b) false allegations of prior abuse by the perpetrator; (c) non-relative caregiver abuse; (d) institutional caregiver abuse; and (e) abuse of male elders by family members. The categories are not mutually exclusive. Many of the reported cases involve murder. This brief note provides vivid accounts, within the five categories, which are offered to detail the actual experiences of the victims, rather than subsuming these victimization experiences within broad and comparatively sterile categorical classifications such as "elder abuse" or "elder neglect." The "grittiness" of these cases yields insight not only with respect to the terror experienced by some of these men, but also of their utter vulnerability, defenselessness, and susceptibility to their own victimization. Especially, it appears, in post-industrial countries where extended family ties often are not robust, social isolation and/or loneliness can be salient contributing aspects to the victimization, particularly in cases involving late-life intimate relationships.

ECONOMIC EXPLOITATION

In Portland, Oregon, forty-three year-old Roxanna Thomas was charged with criminal treatment and theft involving an eighty-two year-old man after an investigation was launched following reports being made of the man's sudden change in attitude toward family members

(James, 2004). Thomas, who worked at a grocery store in which the elderly man shopped, "befriended" him, following which $530,000 worth of the victim's assets either were conveyed outright to Thomas, or her relatives, or the perpetrators were made joint owners of the victim's assets. Officials noted that elder abuse is epidemic in their Washington County community and that economic abuse of elderly men by strangers appears more common than either physical abuse or neglect. The victim ultimately benefited from intervention when he was the subject of an emergency guardianship and his financial accounts were frozen. Other men, ostensibly with little or no contact with relatives, or whose relatives were less vigilant, have not been as fortunate.

Two homeless elderly men, for example, fifty-year-old Kenneth McDavid and seventy-three year-old Paul Vados, both of whom resided in Los Angeles, were found dead after being defrauded out of two million dollars by seventy-two year-old Olga Rutterschmidt and seventy-five year-old Helen Golay (Hong, 2006; Pringle, 2006; Spano, 2006). The women paid for apartments for the men over a period of two years in exchange for the men naming the women as beneficiaries of insurance policies procured by the women. Both men, subsequently, died when involved in separate hit-and-run automobile incidents. The women were arrested when surveillance revealed them talking to several other elderly men who also were observed signing documents provided by the women.

FALSE ALLEGATIONS: VICTIMIZATION BY INTIMATES

In another murder case, twenty-seven year-old Tatjana Edwards, married to seventy-two year-old Gwyn Edwards, was convicted of having murdered her elderly spouse, despite Edwards' false allegations, at trial, of having been physically abused by her husband. The two had met at the London, England massage parlor where Mrs. Edwards worked as a "massage therapist" prior to the marriage. In pronouncing sentence, Judge Geoffrey Rivlin, noting that she had falsely accused her husband of domestic violence and had shown no remorse or contrition, also commented: "You lived with him rather less than two years, during which time you took every penny off him you could, and when you could get no more you took his life away." Edwards used a kitchen knife to stab her husband to death. She was sentenced to a life term, meaning she will have to serve a minimum of twelve years in prison (BBC News, 2006a; BBC News, 2006b; Cheston, 2006; Dodd, 2006; UK News, 2006).

In a similar case, celebrated Canadian, Melissa Friedrich, was a cause célèbre for battered women until she pled guilty to felony charges arising from the victimization of a second elderly male. Friedrich, known as Melissa Stewart at the time she was celebrated, first made headlines in Nova Scotia as an abused woman who had struck back at her allegedly abusive husband, Gordon Stewart. In killing her husband, she gave him a lethal dose of pills, liquor, and rubbing alcohol, and then ran over him with her automobile on a deserted road near Halifax International Airport. Despite the crime's grisliness, Friedrich was featured in Canada's National Film Board documentary, Why Women Kill, as an exponent of battered women's syndrome, and she was given a governmental grant to fund an Ontario hotline for battered women. But she made news, again, following her marriage to eighty-four year-old Robert Friedrich, a man she had met on an Internet dating site, after his children successfully litigated a civil suit alleging that Friedrich had killed their father by administering a lethal overdose of drugs. But Friedrich's story didn't end there. Two years later, amid allegations that she was poisoning hospitalized seventy-three year-old Floridian, Alex Strategos, she was charged with several offenses, including defrauding Canada's social insurance system, after witnesses observed Friedrich forcing Strategos, on his hospital bed, to sign several documents (CBC News, 2006; Leydon, 2005; Thompson, 2005; Tisch, 2006).

NON-RELATIVE CAREGIVERS

Non-hospital and other non-institutionalized settings provide fertile opportunities for abuse because, unlike settings such as retirement homes, assisted living arrangements, and the like, privately arranged care-giving is not regulated. Absent of state regulation and inspection, cases like that of fifty-nine year-old boarding home operator, Dorothea Puente, of Sacramento, California, can go on for years without detection (Nelson, 2002; Wilson, 1997). It may also be that older care-giver women are assumed to be both less inclined and less capable than others of bringing about harm to men, thereby causing them to be more likely to escape suspicion and subsequent detection by law enforcement authorities. In Puente's case, nine bodies of elderly victims, one of whom had been dismembered with his head cut off, were found buried either in Puente's garden or within her boarding home's surrounding premises. Autopsies revealed that all of those murdered had been killed by drug overdoses. Puente's crimes eventually were discovered, but only after she continued to cash the governmental assistance checks of her victims. Puente, however, was convicted only of three murders, not nine, when a male juror refused to believe that she could have been responsible for all of the murders, pointing to an unsophisticated but pervasive belief that women just cannot be as dangerous, or as lethal, as males.

Another California case receiving media attention involved an elderly man brutalized by a burly male home health aide employed by the victim's wife (Gross, 2006). The brutalized man, as he laid on a gurney in a Santa Ana hospital emergency room, repeatedly told the same story of the home health aide's beatings, while the aide, and the victim's wife, insisted that the elderly man had fallen. But the bruises on the man's chest were determined to be the result of having been punched, he had purple bruises all over his body with some of the bruises beginning to fade to yellow, and the man had the bloody outline of a shoe on his leg. Perhaps, in part because the perpetrator was male, a prosecutor was sufficiently convinced to charge the aide with a felony, despite the victim having manifested signs of dementia when interviewed.

INSTITUTIONAL CAREGIVERS

While fertile ground exists for abuse to occur in unlicensed and non-regulated care-giving settings, deterrents imposed by state authority by no means eliminate abuse in licensed institutional settings, as the case of military veteran, Thomas Joyner, illustrates. Fifty-two year-old wheelchair-bound Joyner, a resident of a state run home for veterans located in Barstow, California, had just lit a cigarette when he was accosted by the home's acting administrator, and two employees, who promptly broke Joyner's finger in forcing the cigarette from his hand. Barstow, who had lighted the cigarette in an area of the home referred to as the "olive garden," unknowingly had violated a very recently enacted rule limiting smoking to certain hours and prohibiting smoking in certain areas, such as the olive garden. As noted by Joyner, the three women approached him from behind, held him down, forcibly took the cigarette, breaking the fourth finger on his right hand, and then searched his pockets for more cigarettes. Joyner reported that he said: "Help, you are hurting me . . . Please don't take my cigarettes." Joyner is partially paralyzed, has impaired speech, limited vision and hearing, and he requires assistance in eating, bathing, and taking his medications. Less than two months after his incident, the facility was fined $95,000 in the death of a World War II infantryman and, prior to the infantryman's case, the facility had been ordered to pay fines for the death of a veteran involved in an eating incident, and for the death of another veteran whose diabetes had not been monitored properly. The California Highway Patrol, which investigates crimes occurring on state property, urged prosecutors to file elder abuse charges, in Joyner's case, against the three women (Ingram, 2003). Nursing home resident, seventy-eight year-old Alzheimer's patient, Marshall Rhodes, was beaten at the hands of his institutional caretaker over an eight-month period following which he subsequently died. He had been taken to a hospital after nurses discovered him in his room clothed in a torn and blood-stained sleeping gown. Six months prior to his death, two nursing assistants reported to two supervisors their suspicions that aide Karl Willard was beating Rhodes, but their protestations were rebuffed. Subsequently, Charles B. Kaiser, III, president of the company which operated the home, American Healthcare Management, received the maximum penalty of one year in jail with a fine of $1,000 for having failed to report elder abuse to the state. Additionally, American Healthcare Management, and the home, St. Louis's St. Charles Claywest, also were convicted for failing to report the abuse and each were given maximum fines under Missouri law of $5,000. Karl Willard was found guilty of elder abuse and is serving fifteen years in prison. Prior to the Rhodes' case, American Healthcare Management and Claywest had settled several wrongful death cases out of court. Reportedly, this was the first instance in the State of Missouri in which a nursing home executive was sentenced to jail in a case involving patient abuse (Schremp, 2003).

FAMILY CAREGIVERS

Sixty-eight year-old retiree, plumber, Robert Heitzman, who had suffered debilitating strokes for nearly twenty years, was found dead in the home he shared with his family. He died, lying in excrement, of septic poisoning resulting from infected bedsores due to his being bedridden on the exposed springs of a mattress that was rotting away from his own bodily secretions. At trial, the presiding judge noted that Heitzman's sons could have made a simple phone call to relieve their father of severe suffering. It also was asserted by the prosecutor that the sons failed to do so because the victim was receiving monthly payments of nearly eight hundred dollars in combined Veterans Administration and Social Security payments. Both sons, Jerry and Richard, were convicted of involuntary manslaughter, and sentenced to four-year terms (Pinsky, 1993).

Ralph Dills, formerly lauded as a venerable judge and lawmaker who had served longer than any other politician in California, died on his fifty acre ranch, unable to take a shower when often left alone because feces from his wife's rottweilers littered his bathroom. His wife, fifty-seven year-old Wendi Lewellen, who also was Dills' former non-adopted stepdaughter, had married the ninety-one year-old former lawmaker, less than a year prior to his death, while he already was suffering from Alzheimer's. As reported by family members and confirmed by court and medical records, Lewellen deceived her stepfather by impersonating her deceased mother, thereafter plundering Dills' estate to such an extent that Dills thought he was going broke despite receiving nearly $14,000, monthly, in pensions and Social Security. Allegedly, and prior to the marriage, Lewellen, wielding undue influence, also was the cause of her brother, Leighton Dills, being omitted from the will of Ralph and Elizabeth Dills. Elizabeth Dills, who died in 2000, was Lewellen's natural mother ("Elder Abuse," 2002).

COMMENTS

One theme emerging from the accounts is that many of the victimized men appear isolated, infirm, lonely, and bereft of vigilant family members concerned about their care. One impaired individual who subsequently became a ward had manifested a "sudden change" in attitude toward his family following meeting a younger woman, two individuals were homeless, another married a much younger woman who was a prostitute, and yet another married a woman he met on an Internet dating site. Other victims resided in non-regulated boarding home settings but some victims were domiciled in institutional settings employing staff reminiscent of those portrayed in the movie, One Flew Over the Cuckoo's Nest. On the other hand, several cases involved the complicity of relatives, ostensibly motivated primarily by exploitative economic gain, but one older man was saved from further economic victimization by vigilant family members, whereas another was saved from possible death by witnesses who were vigilant in their observation of his hospital care. Economic motivations were at the heart of many of the cases. Poisoning appeared to be the method of choice in cases involving murder.

In the majority of cases, the victim was infirm prior to being victimized. One individual was sufficiently impaired as to require a court-ordered guardianship over his person and estate, one was partially paralyzed with other infirmities, two were victims of Alzheimer's, and one had suffered debilitating strokes prior to his exploitation. These elderly men were particularly vulnerable, virtually defenseless, and exceedingly suscepti-ble to becoming prey of the unscrupulous.

Many of the unscrupulous perpetrators were women, and some of the women had gone undetected for years despite leaving numerous corpses or individuals victimized by other means in their wake. Given the grisli-ness of their crimes, one is forced to wonder about a prevailing view held by many that women involved in domestic violence simply are not capable of being as lethal as men. Late-life marriages appeared espe-cially implicated in the victimizations.

One theme, not particularly explicated in the accounts, is that per-petrators, institutional and otherwise, tend to receive comparatively meager punishment for their crimes. One individual perpetrator, for example, was even celebrated as a victim of domestic violence, one murderer received a "stiff" sentence of life imprisonment that re-quired a minimum incarceration of only twelve years, another whose vulnerable victim subsequently died will be incarcerated only for fifteen years, and two others received respective terms only of four years. As noted in the accounts, institutional perpetrators are just beginning to be prosecuted.

Another theme not explicitly addressed by the accounts is the role of agency and conservatorships in economic exploitation. An unscru-pulous person designated by an infirm older individual as the elder's attorney-in-fact, or agent, via a power of attorney document, is granted license virtually to loot the elderly person's estate. The only recourse is for a person, or persons, with "standing" recognized by a court, to file suit, following which they must prove that the agent did not act in the best interests of the elder. By then, most often, it is too late. Indeed, in some states, conservators can be appointed without notice to the elder, whereas other states allow a decedent's creditor to become executor of the decedent's estate ("State Needs," 1997; Wisconsin Statutes Chapter 856, 2003-2004). These scenarios leave the door wide open for financial abuse, during life, and afterwards.

REFERENCES

BBC News. (2006a, March 23). Tragic end to unlikely marriage. Retrieved November 25, 2006, http://news.bbc.co.uk/2/hi/uk_news/england/southern_counties/4832588.stm

BBC News. (2006b, March 24). Greedy wife gets life for murder. Retrieved November 25, 2006, from http://news.bbc.co.uk/2/hi/uk_news/england/southern_counties/4841094.stm

CBC News. (2006, March 14). Melissa Friedrich: Internet black widow. Retrieved November 25, 2006, from http://www.cbc.ca/news/background/crime/friedrich.html

Cheston, P. (2006, March 24). Life for gold-digging prostitute who murdered husband of 72. *The Evening Standard*, P1.

Dodd, V. (2006, March 24). Former prostitute found guilty of murdering the husband she had thought was a millionaire. *The Guardian*, P7.

Elder Abuse Suspected in Dills' Marriage. (2002, August 19). *Daily Breeze*, p. A9.

Gross, J. (2006, September 27). Forensic skills seek to uncover hidden patterns of elder abuse. *The New York Times*. Retrieved November 25, 2006, from http://www.nytimes.com/2006/09/27/us/27abuse.html?ex=1164603600&en=c2f944e8d45aa3a9&ei=5070

Hong, P. Y. (2006, September 14). Women plead not guilty in deaths of transients. *The Los Angeles Times*, p. B10.

Ingram, C. (2003, February 26). CHP alleges elder abuse at veterans home: Three employees of a Barstow facility are accused of breaking resident's finger while taking a cigarette from him. *The Los Angeles Times*, p. B8.

James, S. (2004, April 5). Woman arrested after trying to bilk elderly man out of more than a quarter million dollars. Media Information, Washington County, Portland, Oregon, Sheriff's Office. Retrieved November 25, 2006, from http://www.co.washington.or.us/sheriff/media/eld_mill.htm

Leydon, J. (2005, January 13). Internet black widow 'stalked pensioners on the net.' *The Register*. Retrieved November 25, 2006, from http://www.theregister.co.uk/2005/01/13/internet_black_widow/

Nelson, D. (2002, May 2). Valley of death. *Sacramento News and Review*. Retrieved November 25, 2006, from http://www.newsreview.com/sacramento/Content?oid=oid%3A11972

Pinsky, M. I. (1993, March 26). Sons get prison for fatal neglect of their father, courts: Judge cites 'cruelty and depravity' of Huntington Beach brothers who are sentenced to four years for letting parent die of septic poisoning on his rotting mattress. *The Los Angeles Times*, p. 1.

Pringle, P. (2006, August 1). Murder counts filed against pair. *The Los Angeles Times*, p. B1.

Schremp, V. (2003, February 7). Nursing home chief gets one-year sentence; He failed to report elderly abuse. *St. Louis Post-Dispatch*, p. A1.

Spano, J. (2006, August 18). Probe widens in transient deaths: Two women accused of running over two men to collect death benefits may have targeted three others, police say. *The Los Angeles Times*, p. B1.

Spano, J. (2006, August 30). Arraignment in killings postponed: Two women accused of slaying transients for insurance money are to enter pleas Sept. 13. *The Los Angeles Times*, p. B4.

State needs better oversight of professional conservators; unwanted takeover of O.C. senior's affairs raises concern. *The Los Angeles Times* (Orange County Edition), p. 8.

Thompson, J. (2005, January 12). Police say woman victimized companion. *St. Petersburg Times Online*. Retrieved November 25, 2006, from http://www.sptimes.com/2005/01/12/Tampabay/Police_say_woman_vict.shtml

Tisch, C. (2006, March 15). Scamming woman gets 5-year term. *St. Petersburg Times Online* Retrieved November 25, 2006, from http://www.sptimes.com/2005/03/15/Northpinellas/Scamming_woman_gets_5.shtml

UK News. (2006, March 23). Estonian prostitute accused of murdering elderly husband. Retrieved November 25, 2006, from http://www.lse.co.uk/ShowStory.asp?story=EB723232W&news_headline=estonian_proStitue_accused_of_murdering

Wilson, W. (1997, September 10). Puente's conviction reaffirmed but misconduct charge will be probed. *The Sacramento Bee*, p. B1.

Wisconsin Statutes Chapter 856, Wisc. Stat. §§ 856-07(2) (2003-2004).

doi:10.1300/J084v19n01_07

Identifying and Working
with Older Male Victims
of Abuse in England

Jacki Pritchard, MA

SUMMARY. The abuse of men is still very much a taboo subject, so identifying older men who have been abused in childhood or adulthood can be very difficult. This paper discusses the problems in identifying older male victims by drawing on the findings of two research projects. Statistical evidence is presented regarding the victims and the abuse they have experienced. It is argued that in general resources are not readily available to facilitate disclosure or to help men through the healing process. An example of good practice is presented by discussing the work

---

Jacki Pritchard is an Independent Researcher, Consultant and Trainer in Social Care, and an Independent Social Worker (General Social Care Registration Number: 1058524).

Address correspondence to: Jacki Pritchard Ltd, Units G9 and G10, The Globe Business Centre, Penistone Road, Sheffield, South Yorkshire, S6 3AE, England (E-mail: jacki.Pritchard@btconnect.com).

Please note the facts presented and views expressed in this article are those of the author and not necessarily those of the Joseph Rowntree Foundation.

The author acknowledges that this paper could never have been written if victims and workers had not willingly participated in and contributed to the two research projects. She also is indebted to everyone who has been a member of the Beyond Existing groups during the past six years. Finally, very special thanks to Mr. Ron Haimes.

[Haworth co-indexing entry note]: "Identifying and Working with Older Male Victims of Abuse in England." Pritchard, Jacki. Co-published simultaneously in *Journal of Elder Abuse & Neglect*™ (The Haworth Maltreatment & Trauma Press®, an imprint of The Haworth Press, Inc.) Vol. 19, No. 1/2, 2007, pp. 109-127; and: *Abuse of Older Men* (ed: Jordan I. Kosberg) The Haworth Maltreatment & Trauma Press®, an imprint of The Haworth Press, Inc., 2007, pp. 109-127. Single or multiple copies of this article are available for a fee from The Haworth Document Delivery Service [1-800-HAWORTH, 9:00 a.m. - 5:00 p.m. (EST). E-mail address: docdelivery@haworthpress.com].

undertaken with an older man through group work. doi:10.1300/J084

v19n01_08 *[Article copies available for a fee from The Haworth Document Delivery Service: 1-800-HAWORTH. E-mail address: <docdelivery@haworth press.com> Website: <http://www.HaworthPress.com> © 2007 by The Haworth Press, Inc. All rights reserved.]*

KEYWORDS. Male victims, elder abuse, abuse identification and monitoring, disclosure, healing process, group work, creative writing

INTRODUCTION

The abuse of older men is still very much a taboo subject in England. It is hard to get society as a whole to accept the fact that men are abused in similar ways to female victims of abuse. Men tend to be seen as perpetrators of abuse rather than victims. Workers in the field of health and social care also can fail to recognise that men are vulnerable to abuse; hence they may not be identified as victims and their needs are not met. The purpose of this paper is to consider how older men who have been abused (whether in childhood or adulthood) are being identified and what work is being undertaken with them to meet their needs. This paper will draw from two research projects plus work which is being undertaken in support groups for male victims.[1]

BACKGROUND TO THE RESEARCH PROJECTS

Before discussing the needs of male victims of abuse, it is necessary to explain how the two research projects came into being. In 1997 funding was secured from the Joseph Rowntree Foundation for a project entitled *The Needs of Older Women: Services for Victims of Elder Abuse.* The project was undertaken in three social services departments in the North of England[2] and its main aims were to:

1. Identify women who were victims of elder abuse.
2. Carry out a small study to identify the extent to which victims of elder abuse have also experienced abuse earlier in their lives.
3. Identify the types of abuse experienced (in childhood and adulthood).
4. Identify the needs of victims.
5. Consider what resources or services should be provided for victims.

Consequently, the project involved both a quantitative study and a qualitative study. The monitoring systems developed for the quantitative study will be discussed in detail below. One of the methods used for the qualitative part of the study was to run focus groups for service users. I spent a lot of time in care homes and day centres for older people and became known as "the abuse lady." People understood what I was trying to achieve through the project and this had a very positive effect in that victims would voluntarily come to talk to me about their experiences, knowing that they would be listened to and taken seriously (i.e., believed). Hence, what developed from the project was the concept of giving victims "permission to speak."

The focus groups were intended for female service users, but men started to ask if they could also attend, which they did with the agreement of the women. At the same time, men approached me individually to ask if they could tell me about their experiences of abuse. It was at this early stage in the project that it was decided to broaden the focus of inquiry to include older men who had experienced abuse.

The project ran until the year 2000 when the findings for the women were published (Pritchard, 2000). In the following year the findings regarding male victims were published (Pritchard, 2001c). I continued to monitor the statistics in two of the social services departments for a further two years, which are presented in this paper as part of the original project.

An important development after the project officially finished was that the Joseph Rowntree Foundation agreed to fund a further pilot project for a year. A need which had been identified by both male and female victims was to meet other people who had experienced abuse. The pilot project set up support groups for both men and women who had experienced abuse either in childhood or adulthood. The pilot, which ran for a year, proved to be very beneficial to the victims who wanted their groups to continue. Funding was secured and the groups developed into an organisation called Beyond Existing (Pritchard, 2003). The organisation has since broadened its responsibility to work with any vulnerable adult (i.e., anyone over 18 years of age), not just older victims. Some of the work undertaken with older men will be explained later in this paper.

Just as the original research project was completed, the Department of Health (DH) launched the guidance, *No Secrets: Guidance on Developing and Implementing Multi-Agency Policies and Procedures to Protect Vulnerable Adults from Abuse,* under the Local Authority and Social Services Act 1970 (DH 2000a). A Circular issued from the Department of Health (DH 2000b: Health Service/Local Authority Circular HSC 2000/007, p. 2) stated: "Directors of Social Services will be expected to ensure that the local multi-agency codes of practice are developed and implemented by 31st October 2001."

Six years after the launch of *No Secrets,* I decided to undertake a follow-on research project to see how things had developed in regard to whether services have been meeting the needs of victims of abuse. There have been many diverse responses to the guidance and it is very evident that adult abuse is dealt with very differently by social services and other key agencies (such as Police, Health, Commission for Social Care Inspection) around the UK. The main objective of the new research project is to consider how two social services departments have responded to the DH guidance since 2000 and to evaluate whether victims' needs are being met. As in the original project, I wanted to give victims a voice. Thus, the second project was started in April 2006 and, at the time of writing this paper, has been running for 6 months. Current statistics and findings from one social services department will be presented in this paper.[3]

IDENTIFYING MALE VICTIMS

It has already been stated that society still finds it hard to believe that men can be abused. This is a sad reflection when people like Steinmetz and Straus had highlighted the problem in America during the 1970s and continued to do so into the Millennium (Steinmetz, 1978; Straus, Gelles, & Steinmetz, 1980; Straus & Gelles, 1986; Straus, 1999). In order to raise awareness, it is imperative that we disclose how many men are abused; that is, we need the evidence. In 1996, the British Crime Survey (Home Office, 1996), which concluded that men were just as likely as women to be victims of domestic violence, found an increase in domestic attacks on men by women. The survey determined that 4.2% of men indicated that they had been assaulted by a partner in 1995. Nearly a decade later, the British Crime Survey broadened its focus to include domestic violence, sexual assault and stalking (Walby & Allen, 2004). Consequently, the findings are much more detailed. There were two key findings regarding domestic violence. First, partner abuse (non-sexual) was more likely to have been experienced since the age of 16 by women (28%) and men (18%) than other forms of abuse. Second, a half of women (50%) and a third of men (35%) who had experienced intimate violence since the age of 16 had experienced more than one type of intimate violence in that time (Finney, 2006).

When the original project was set up in 1997, few social services departments had sophisticated monitoring systems. The project set up monitoring systems in the three departments in order to collect data regarding all adult abuse referrals. Monitoring forms were designed in such a way to analyse information concerning victims, abusers, types of abuse perpetrated, and action taken.

An ongoing problem in the field of research is that researchers utilise different definitions of abuse. An objective of this research was to see how older people defined not only their own abuse but also abuse in general. However, the definition which was adopted for the project was based on the DH definition from 1993: "Abuse may be described as physical, sexual, psychological or financial. It may be intentional or unintentional or the result of neglect. It causes harm to the older person, either temporarily or over a period of time" (DH, 1993, p. 3).

For the second project, the DH definition from *No Secrets* was adopted (DH 2000a, p. 9):

> Abuse may consist of a single act or repeated acts. It may be physical, verbal psychological, it may be an act of neglect or an omission to act, or it may occur when a vulnerable person is persuaded to enter into a financial or sexual transaction to which he or she has not consented, or cannot consent. Abuse can occur in any relationship and may result in significant harm to, or exploitation of, the person subjected to it.

Since the advent of *No Secrets,* more local areas have developed monitoring systems, but the levels of sophistication differ tremendously. Many Adult Protection Committees produce annual reports which are helpful to establish trends regarding incidence. Action on Elder Abuse has produced an insightful report regarding the findings of The Adult Protection Analysis Project which aimed "to investigate and develop ways of reporting upon, and subsequently analysing data, obtained from Local Authorities and other key parties, under Adult Protection policies developed through *No Secrets* Guidance. The intention was to establish a national recording system for incidents of adult abuse . . ." (Action on Elder Abuse, 2006, p. 6).

However, we have to remember that many managers and workers currently feel overwhelmed with paperwork and the reality is that they can forget to complete monitoring forms, so statistics are not totally reliable. Other problems relate to the fact that many men will not speak out about what is happening to them and, even if they do, very often they are not believed. Thus, identifying male victims of abuse can be extremely difficult. Hopefully, knowledge regarding prevalence of elder abuse in the UK will increase in the future as the UK National Prevalence Study of the Mistreatment and Abuse of Older People is undertaken in 2007. The study started in August 2005, after concern was expressed by Members of Parliament who formed the Health Select Committee regarding the lack of knowledge about elder abuse (McCreadie et al., 2006).

What follows are the findings regarding older men from the original project, together with findings from the first six months of the current project.

NUMBER OF OLDER MALE VICTIMS

In the original project an older man was defined as a male over the age of 60 years. To become consistent with how older people are now defined across the UK, the new project defines an older man as being over 65 years.

Original Project

Table 1 presents the statistics from the original research project. Through the three stages of the project, older men consistently constituted 15% of all vulnerable adult/adult abuse referrals.

As seen in Table 2, older people formed the largest group of vulnerable adults to be referred regarding abuse (63%). Of the 269 older people who were abused, 25% were men, which is a very significant number.

TABLE 1. Referrals–Vulnerable Adults and Older People

	Vulnerable Adults	Older People	Older Men	Older Men as % of Vulnerable Adults
Stage 1	186	126	29	15.6%
Stage 2	258	171	39	15.1%
Stage 3	430	269	67	15.6%

(End of Monitoring Stage 1–March 1999; Stage 2–March 2000; Stage 3–March 2002)

Table 3 presents the age distribution of those men whose ages were known; they ranged between 60 and 102 years:

Current Project

The new research project has found similar trends in the first six months of its quantitative study. However, during the nine years from when the original research monitoring systems were set up, systems have become more detailed and Greenflat social services department has developed a very comprehensive monitoring system. As soon as a referral (often now called an 'alert') is received, managers are expected to complete a monitoring form which is then electronically submitted to the Adult Protection Coordinator. What has been evident is that it is not just individuals who have been identified as victims of abuse; groups of residents in care homes also have been identified.

So in a six month period, 142 cases have been referred that include individuals and groups of residents. Table 4 shows that 67 of these referrals were regarding older people (47%), 23 of which were relating to individual or groups of older men (16.2%).

TABLE 2. Abused Adults

Vulnerable adults	(over 18 years)	430	
Older people	(over 60 years)	269	(63% of vulnerable adults)
Older people: female		202	(47% of vulnerable adults)
Older people: male		67	(15% of vulnerable adults)

TABLE 3. Known Ages of Male Victims

Age	Number of Male Victims
60-64	4
65-69	12
70-74	8
75-79	11
80-84	9
85-89	9
90-94	1
95-99	0
100+	1

TABLE 4. Greenflat Adult Abuse Referrals (First Six Months)

Vulnerable adults	(over 18 years)	142	
Older people cases	(over 65 years)	67	(47% of vulnerable adults)
Older people: individual females		43	(30% of vulnerable adults)
Older people: individual males		21	(15% of vulnerable adults)
Older people: groups of residents in care homes		3	(2% of vulnerable adults)

The ages of the 21 male victims ranged from 65 to 94 years, and those 80 to 84 comprised the largest age category of abused men (N = 8). It also was found that 13 of the 21 abused men were aged 80 and older.

TYPES OF ABUSE EXPERIENCED

Prior to 2000, the DH's definition of abuse included five categories of abuse (physical, sexual, psychological, financial/material, and neglect) but, after the introduction of *No Secrets,* **discriminatory abuse** was added as a sixth category (DH, 2000a, p. 9).

No Secrets also defines institutional abuse as:

> Neglect and poor professional practice also need to be taken into account. This may take the form of isolated incidents of poor or unsatisfactory professional practice, at one end of the spectrum, through to pervasive ill treatment or gross misconduct at the other. Repeated instances of poor care may be an indication of more serious problems and this is sometimes referred to as **institutional abuse.** (DH, 2000, p. 10)

Both discriminatory abuse and institutional abuse are defined as separate categories of abuse; giving the project two categories of abuse which were not defined as such in the original project, affecting the analysis for the quantitative study of the current project.

This section only presents statistics from the quantitative studies, as data for the current project (concerning types of abuse via qualitative research) have not yet been obtained in depth and would not be meaningful. Telephone and face-to-face interviews have been undertaken with managers and workers involved with the male victims. I also have had access to minutes of strategy meetings and reports prepared for case conferences. Table 5 shows that in the original quantitative study, financial and physical abuse were the most common forms of abuse experienced by older men.

Even in the early stages of the current project it is easy to see from the data collected that monitoring forms are being completed in very different ways. It has been stated already that for abuse taking place in care homes, some monitoring forms are being completed for individual victims, whereas others are being completed for groups of residents. It was found that nine of the 21 older men (43%) referred as victims of abuse were living in residential settings, eight men were abused by a paid member of staff, and three of the men were victims of institutional abuse. One man was abused by a female service user with whom he was having a relationship, and this could be deemed to be an example of

TABLE 5. Types of Elder Abuse Experienced by Older Men
(Original Project)

Category of Abuse	Number of Male Victims
Financial	35
Physical	33
Emotional	19
Neglect	10
Sexual	4

TABLE 6. Types of Elder Abuse Experienced by Older Men
(April to September 2006)

Category of Abuse	Number of Individual Male Victims
Emotional	9
Physical	8
Neglect	8
Financial	6
Discriminatory	1
Institutional	3
Sexual	0

Category of Abuse	Number of Groups of Male Residents
Neglect	2
Institutional	1

domestic violence. Table 6 shows the types of abuse experienced by men in the current project.

It is very clear that neglect is the most common form of abuse experienced by older men in the current project. During interviews with workers it became obvious that many of the cases which reported physical or emotional abuse on the monitoring form were actually cases of neglect. Currently, neglect of an adult is not a criminal offence in England. This will change in 2007 when the offence of Neglect and Ill Treatment will be introduced under the Mental Capacity Act 2005. When gross physical neglect is taking place, it can be easier to identify but often neglect (especially emotional neglect) is carried out in very subtle ways and subsequently it is harder to recognise. Proving neglect in child abuse cases is very hard, indeed, and when dealing with adults, workers may 'fail to grasp the nettle' because of the lack of support to date from the criminal justice system (Pritchard, 2001b).

In both research projects it has been evident that older men are victims of domestic violence, which is a form of adult abuse. In England there has been much debate about whether domestic violence should be addressed under adult protection procedures, as distinct specialisms have developed over the years. Dangerous practices may result, if professionals are too precious about their own roles and fail to communicate with workers within other specialisms. In Greenflat the Adult Protection procedures have been used when men have been abused by their wives.

When considering who abused the men, it has been evident in both projects that a wide range of relationships have existed between victims and their abusers. In the original project, the most common abusers were wife (12), resident/service user (8), daughter (6), son (5), residential staff group (4), and friend (4). In the current project, wives and residential staff are again presenting as the most common abusers: individual care worker (7), residential staff group (5), and wife (5).

PROBLEMS IN IDENTIFYING MEN

There are a number of factors which make it very difficult to obtain a true picture of how many older men are abused. It is hard for victims of abuse to disclose their experiences; a common fear is that they will not be believed. This can be an even greater obstacle for men, as they are often seen as perpetrators rather than victims. Many people cannot visualise a man being abused. There is a need to understand that abuse is often carried out in very subtle ways. Neglect, which seems to be a common form of abuse for men in Greenflat, can be incredibly difficult to identify. Workers in all settings need to have their awareness raised but, in addition, they need to be trained in depth to recognise the indicators of abuse.

CASE: MR. BRUCE (AGE 73)[4]

Types of Abuse Alleged: Physical, Emotional and Neglect

Mr. Bruce had been known to mental health services because of having Recurrent Depressive Disorder. He was being monitored under the care programming approach; support was being offered by a community psychiatric nurse. An abuse alert was made by the Consultant Psychiatrist after she had seen Mr. Bruce with his wife in clinic. Mrs. Bruce had openly admitted she had stopped giving Mr. Bruce his medication because she believed the Consultant was poisoning her husband. Instead she was giving him St. John's Wart. There had been a history of Mrs. Bruce stopping her husband's medication and repeated failure to keep hospital appointments. Mr. Bruce had other health problems: he was deaf and had just been diagnosed as having prostrate cancer. The Consultant had concerns about "severe psychological abuse" and the fact that Mrs. Bruce had repeatedly made complaints against other Consultants which resulted in her obstructing the making and keeping of appointments for her husband. It was very difficult for any professional to see or speak to Mr. Bruce on his own.

Crucial questions arise for older men: Where can they go for help? Who will take them seriously? What advice and support is available? Another issue which has been highlighted in Greenflat is that the majority of male victims have cognitive problems and therefore have been incapable of accessing help for themselves. Some victims who have a form of dementia may be able to talk about what is happening to them, but another dilemma is whether they will be taken seriously if and when they do disclose. Whether living in the community or in a residential setting, these men are often extremely vulnerable and isolated because of their own lack of knowledge about how and where to access help. Also, they can lack help and support from others.

CASE: JOE (AGE 81)

Types of Abuse Alleged: Financial

Joe was in the advanced stages of Alzheimer's disease and lived alone. His daughter lived in another city and only visited occasionally. Joe refused all services. Julie, the next door neighbour, became Joe's primary carer and had access to his bank account, credit cards, PIN numbers, etc. Joe's daughter discovered large amounts of money were unaccounted for and reported this to social services who advised her to go to the police. Julie was interviewed but denied that she had been stealing from Joe. The police said that nothing more could be done, as Joe could not clarify whether he had given consent for Julie to have the money which had gone missing.

There is also the issue regarding police commitment to working with victims who are cognitively impaired. In 2002, the Home Office Guidance *Achieving Best Evidence* was implemented and clearly advocates that all vulnerable adults have the right to justice (Home Office, 2002). Police forces are expected to try to gather the "best evidence" they can when an adult has communication difficulties; the adult should not be written off as "not being a credible witness." The use of video interviewing is encouraged. Police practices around the UK differ tremendously. In Greenflat the social services department regularly contacts the police, but to date there have been few successful investigations (in obtaining good evidence) and subsequent prosecutions when older men have been the victims.

For those in residential settings, residents may feel like they are "trapped" or "imprisoned." It is easy to forget that some older men have no living relatives and friends with whom to talk about their abuse. Many older people are placed in residential care settings and only have annual reviews (sometimes by an unknown social worker or reviewing officer). Other residents are self-funding and may never receive visits from those representing a statutory agency. Who is going to identify these victims? Residents also can be fearful of the consequences of speaking out, especially if the abuser is a member of staff. Will the other members of staff believe them, or might staff members make life very difficult for the resident alleging abuse?

Thus, there are many questions about the feasibility of men being able to disclose. They may be hampered by their own physical and mental health problems, together with a lack of useful systems to facilitate disclosure and help. Out of the 23 alerts regarding older men, only two men were self-referred, and five cases were reported by family members. The remainder were reported by paid workers who included social workers, support workers in housing associations, managers and workers in care homes, and inspectors from the regulatory body Commission of Social Care Inspection.

CASE: STEPHEN (AGE 83)

Type of Abuse Alleged: Neglect

Stephen was admitted to hospital from a nursing home with acute confusion and a painful knee. An abuse investigation took place after Stephen's nephew told the hospital social worker about his concerns regarding Stephen's care in the home. Family members had recently found Stephen sitting alone in the dining room with food in his lap. The nephew described Stephen as being "so dehydrated he was unable to open his mouth or speak" and said that Stephen had not been given his prescribed medication for five days. The nephew also found that Stephen's hearing aid and walking stick were missing; in his bedroom, his bed had been moved up against the wall so that other residents' walking frames and a wheelchair could be stored in there. There was no duvet on the bed or hangers in the wardrobe. When investigated, it was found that no care plans had been developed in relation to specific aspects of need and there was no documentary evidence of any ongoing nursing evaluation relating to Stephen's physical or mental health needs.

What has happened more in Greenflat during the last six months is that managers and care workers themselves have been reporting abuse in their own homes. This is extremely positive and must, in part, be due to the work which has been undertaken by the Adult Protection Coordinator who has been visiting homes in the independent sector to raise awareness about abuse and the Coordinator's role. In addition, three half-day conferences were organised by social services to raise awareness about adult abuse which were offered free of charge to organisations within the independent and voluntary sectors.

WORKING WITH MALE VICTIMS

It is clear that the statistics regarding older male victims are a gross underestimation of the real prevalence. However, for those who are identified, the question of "How can they be helped?" must be raised. In general, workers often do not feel very confident about working with abuse. They often are worried about "getting it wrong" when identifying and investigating cases, and few workers are trained to offer long-term skilled therapeutic help. It is very important that any male victim be offered the chance to work through what has happened to him; that is, he needs to be able to talk about what has taken place and to understand why it has happened and that he is not to blame. It is never possible to predict the length of the healing process, but it is vital that long-term support is offered. The following is an example of how such support can be provided to male victims in the Beyond Existing program.

BEYOND EXISTING

Beyond Existing came into being initially as a pilot study within the Churchtown area of the original project, and then developed into a voluntary organisation. As mentioned previously, one of the key needs of male victims of abuse is to have somewhere to go to be able to disclose their abuse and to have the opportunity to go through the healing process. The pilot study was set up in order to meet these needs by offering support through group work. The work of Beyond Existing has been written up elsewhere (Pritchard, 2003; Pritchard & Sainsbury, 2004), but it is important to summarize how the groups have been able to meet the needs of older male victims.

Elder Abuse and Past Abuse

It was found that four of the 12 men who had been part of the qualitative study, in Churchtown social services department, went on to be involved in the pilot study. All had been victims of elder abuse, but two of them had also experienced abuse earlier in their lives (either as a child and/or in earlier adulthood), as shown in Table 7.

A key need for many older people is to address issues from abuse experienced either in childhood or earlier in adulthood (Pritchard, 2001a). It is hard enough for men to discuss their abuse in general, but an added problem for older men is that they were brought up in an era when people were not encouraged to talk about their problems and to vent their feelings. Thus, it can sometimes be incredibly hard for men to verbalise what has happened to them. However, the work which has been done through Beyond Existing groups clearly demonstrates that men can benefit from participating in group work.

TABLE 7. Recent and Past Abuse

Victim	Types of Elder Abuse	Child Abuse	Domestic Violence
Bert (68)	FN	NO	NO
William (79)	PFNS	NO	NO
Jim (76)	PEFS	NO	YES
Vernon (80)	N	YES	YES

Key: P = physical; E = emotional; F = financial; N = neglect; S = sexual

Many different types of groups have been facilitated during the past 6 years. Some men have attended "mixed" groups; that is, they have been in groups with female victims. One such group included men and women who had been sexually abused. Local professionals cynically suggested it would never succeed, but in fact it worked exceedingly well. William was one person who gained tremendous help and support from a female victim, Lilian, who had also been part of the original research project. William's sexual abuse included rape by his male carer; Lilian had been sexually abused by her brother in childhood.

In April 2004, a group was set up specifically for men over 18 years of age. This has been an open group, so membership has changed during this time. All the men who have attended have experienced sexual abuse in childhood. One older man, Ron, attended regularly through the two years and has now worked through the healing process. With Ron's permission I am able to share his story to illustrate the work which can be achieved with older male victims.

Ron

Ron, who is 63 years of age, was a victim of child abuse. He was grossly neglected by his parents and sexually abused by two men who targeted and groomed him. The abuses he experienced have affected his mental health throughout his adult life. He is currently supported by a social worker from the local community mental health team. He suffers from acute anxiety and depression which has led to him to be unable to go out of the house on his own. Ron also has various physical health problems. His social worker referred Ron to Beyond Existing when the men's group was being set up, and Ron attended monthly meetings regularly for two years.

The general aim of Beyond Existing is to provide practical and emotional support, but it is made very clear to members that the main objective is to offer a therapeutic environment (that is, to help them through the healing process). For some victims, group work does not help to facilitate this process, they need one-to-one work. For others, group work is the appropriate intervention to address abuse issues.

A variety of methods are used in the groups: group discussion, individual work with the aid of one of the group facilitators, group exercises, working with another member of the group, role playing, writing in a journal, writing poetry, and drawing. The creative writing has been one of the most successful ways of working with both men and women; many of them have written journals, stories or poems (Pritchard & Sainsbury, 2004). The writing helps victims to re-live the earlier abuse, vent feelings about the abuser and others, express current feelings, explain current fears and problems, and convey hopes for the future.

Ron was extremely nervous when he attended the first group meeting and admitted months later he never thought he would be able to get into the meeting room. However, once he had met the other men (all of whom had who had also experienced child sexual abuse), he felt he could talk about his own experiences.

Ron described vividly the dreadful conditions in which he lived with his parents. He regularly talked about the terrible state of his clothes, shoes, the dirt on his own body and the fact that he was always starving because he was not fed. His parents left him for long periods of time whilst they drank excessively in the local public houses. Ron was extremely bitter about how he had never been cared for by his parents, but he blamed his mother rather than his father for this. He felt very bitter towards his mother who spent a great deal of time in hospitals because of her physical and mental health problems. Ron also talked openly about the fact that his father was a paedophile who targeted young girls.

From a very early age, Ron had hated going home to an empty, cold house; he spent a lot of time wandering the streets in the local community. He was befriended by a man who was deaf and had no speech. This man gave Ron money (which he desperately needed for food) in return for sex. Ron was also sexually abused by the man's friend who visited the house.

A variety of methods was used to help Ron through the healing process. Once he had gained his confidence, he openly talked about the abuse and could recount in detail the incidents which had stayed in his mind. He also eventually talked about his recurring nightmares about sexual acts he had been forced to perform with the two men. Ron was reluctant at first to use drawing as a medium for expression, but after about a year he did start to draw his life pattern. However, the over-riding factor in the work undertaken with Ron was his poetry. He has always been gifted with the skills to produce poetry and this helped him through the healing process. In between meetings he would write poems and then bring them to the meetings.

The poems Ron wrote gave clear insight into what he was struggling with in between the meetings and we were able to work on these issues with him. Ron had recurring nightmares about the sexual acts he was forced to engage in. In the following, Ron's two poems clearly portray the torment he experienced when he went to sleep.

NIGHTMARE

Last night as I slept
Into a tormented mind I crept,
What I witnessed there,
Turned my bones to jelly, greyed my hair.
Acid rain poured down, blistered his skin,
This man must have committed a dreadful sin.
With Imps and Goblins, by the score,
Moans and groans from the graveyard floor.
Demons appear carrying buckets of gore.
Then after listening to the Devil's roar,
I did not want to stay there anymore,
So with a thumping heart, aching head,
I awoke in a tangle, at the bottom of the bed.

IN ONE EAR OUT THE OTHER

My mind shut down, goes to sleep
Gets rid of the memories I long to keep
I am slow you might say
For in the house I mostly stay

My mind is deaf and can be blind
But then again I won't have to mind
All I can do is hope one day
That the mists that fog my mind will lift and blow away

The final task Ron undertook before the group finished was to write a letter to his two abusers. The letter could not be sent (as it is not known whether the men are dead or alive), but it was important for Ron to tell the men how he felt about what they had done to him. It is not appropriate to reproduce the letter here, as it is something private to Ron, but he did share it within the group. One of the major achievements for Ron has been that he no longer blames himself for the abuse. Throughout adulthood he had felt he was a bad person because he had taken money for sex. The writing of the letter firmly acknowledged that the two men were responsible for Ron being a victim of child sexual abuse.

CONCLUSION

We shall never know the true prevalence of abuse, as there will always be victims who are fearful to speak out. However, there is no doubt that the abuse of older men is an important social issue that still remains well hidden. The findings of the two research projects discussed in this paper clearly show that a significant number of older men have experienced abuse in childhood and adulthood, but help may not be readily available or consistent. This is because male victims are not systematically identified due to a lack of awareness about their vulnerability, the lack of skills to identify different forms of abuse, or the failure to offer them an opportunity to speak out. Male victims need to be offered the chance to disclose and heal; therefore, organisations across all the sectors (statutory, voluntary and independent) must begin to provide adequate training for their workers to identify male victims of abuse and to also provide them with appropriate resources.

NOTES

1. The word 'victim' rather than survivor will be used in this paper.
2. The three departments were given fictitious names in research publications to keep anonymity of the victims; these were known as Churchtown, Millfield and Tallyborough.
3. The department has been given the fictitious name **Greenflat**.
4. Fictitious names have been used to keep anonymity of victims.

REFERENCES

Action on Elder Abuse. (2006). *Adult protection data collection and reporting requirements*. London: AEA.
Department of Health. (1993). *No longer afraid: The safeguard of older people in domestic settings*. London: HMSO.
Department of Health. (2000a). *No secrets: Guidance on developing and implementing multi-agency policies and procedures to protect vulnerable adults from abuse*. London: DH.

Department of Health. (2000b). "No secrets" Guidance on developing multi-agency policies and procedures to protect vulnerable adults from abuse. Health Service/ Local Authority Circular HSC 2000/007.

Finney, A. (2006). *Domestic violence, sexual assault and stalking: Findings from the 2004/05 British Crime Survey.* London: Home Office Online Report 12/06.

Home Office. (2002). *Achieving best evidence in criminal proceedings: Guidance for vulnerable of intimidated witnesses.* London: Home Office Communication Directorate.

Home Office. (1996). *Domestic violence. Home Office Research Study 191.* London: HMSO.

McCreadie, C., O'Keeffe M., Manthorpe, J., Tinker, A., Doyle, M., Hills, A., & Erens, B. (2006). First steps: The UK prevalence study of the mistreatment and abuse of older people. *The Journal of Adult Protection, 8*(3), 4-11.

Pritchard, J. (2001a). Abuse in earlier life. In J. Pritchard (Ed.), *Good practice with vulnerable adults* (pp. 164-184). London: Jessica Kingsley Publishers.

Pritchard, J. (2001b). Neglect: Not grasping the nettle and hiding behind choice. In J. Pritchard (Ed.), *Good practice with vulnerable adult* (pp. 224-244). London: Jessica Kingsley Publishers.

Pritchard, J. (2001c). *Male victims of abuse: Their experiences and needs.* London: Jessica Kingsley Publishers.

Pritchard, J. (2000). *The needs of older women: Services for victims of elder abuse and other abuse.* Bristol: The Policy Press.

Pritchard, J. (2003). *Support groups for older people who have been abused: Beyond existing.* London: Jessica Kingsley Publishers.

Pritchard, J. & Sainsbury, E. (2004). *Can you read me?: Creative writing with child and adult victims of abuse.* London: Jessica Kingsley Publishers.

Steinmetz, S.K. (1978). The battered husband syndrome. *Victimology, 2,* 499-509.

Straus, M. (1999). The controversy over domestic violence by women: A methodological, theoretical and sociology of science analysis. In X.B. Arriaga & A. Oskamp (Eds.), *Violence in intimate relationships.* Thousand Oaks: Sage.

Straus, M.A., & Gelles, R.J. (1986). Societal change and change in family violence from 1975 to 1985 as revealed by two national surveys. *Journal of Marriage and the Family, 48,* 465-479.

Straus, M.A., Gelles, R.J., & Steinmetz, S.K. (1980). *Behind closed doors: Violence in the American family.* Garden City, NY: Anchor.

Walby, S., & Allen, J. (2004 March). *Domestic violence, sexual assault and stalking: Findings from the British Crime Survey. Home Research Study 276.* London: Home Office Research, Development and Statistics Directorate.

doi:10.1300/J084v19n01_08

Gendered Policies and Practices that Increase Older Men's Risk of Elder Mistreatment

Edward H. Thompson Jr., PhD
William Buxton, BA
P. Casey Gough, BA
Cara Wahle, BA

SUMMARY. We aim to detail some of the ways that social policy and gendered practices put older men at risk of elder mistreatment. Research on the abuse and neglect that older adults experience has often focused on the characteristics of the victims and the dynamics within families, emphasizing factors such as the likelihood of an intergenerational cycle of violence, substance abuse and dependency, and older men's financial status as key risks in elder abuse. The effect on men from this type of analysis is that elder mistreatment remains an individual or family problem rather than being viewed as a larger societal concern. This article challenges

Edward H. Thompson, Jr. is Director of the Gerontology Studies Program and Professor of Sociology, Department of Sociology & Anthropology, College of the Holy Cross. William Buxton, P. Casey Gough, and Cara Wahle were sociology majors completing their last year of undergraduate work at the College of the Holy Cross.

Address correspondence to: Edward H. Thompson, Jr., Chair, Department of Sociology and Anthropology, College of Holy Cross, 1 College Street, Worcester, MA 01610-2395 (E-mail: ethompson@holycross.edu).

[Haworth co-indexing entry note]: "Gendered Policies and Practices that Increase Older Men's Risk of Elder Mistreatment." Thompson Jr., Edward H. et al. Co-published simultaneously in *Journal of Elder Abuse & Neglect*™ (The Haworth Maltreatment & Trauma Press®, an imprint of The Haworth Press, Inc.) Vol. 19, No. 1/2, 2007, pp. 129-151; and: *Abuse of Older Men* (ed: Jordan I. Kosberg) The Haworth Maltreatment & Trauma Press®, an imprint of The Haworth Press, Inc., 2007, pp. 129-151. Single or multiple copies of this article are available for a fee from The Haworth Document Delivery Service [1-800-HAWORTH, 9:00 a.m. - 5:00 p.m. (EST). E-mail address: docdelivery@haworthpress.com].

129

the individualistic focus by outlining the importance of societal forces affecting older men's risk of mistreatment. doi:10.1300/J084v19n01_09

[Article copies available for a fee from The Haworth Document Delivery Service: 1-800-HAWORTH. E-mail address: <docdelivery@haworthpress.com> Website: <http://www.HaworthPress.com> © 2007 by The Haworth Press, Inc. All rights reserved.]

KEYWORDS. Masculinity, old men, elder mistreatment, abuse, neglect, vulnerability

INTRODUCTION

Mistreatment of an older person, whether in a family setting, institutional caregiving arrangement, or on the street, remains a largely ignored *and* hidden social problem (Wolf, 2000). Although it is not an "epidemic running rampant through society" (Johnson, 1991, p. 5), perhaps one older adult in sixteen has been abused. But this is an estimate. The abuse and neglect older adults experience is more often managed quietly and privately. It may not be obvious even to the victims. Thus, the problem lies below a threshold of public scrutiny.

For these and other reasons, the one-to-sixteen ratio understates the number of mistreated older adults, particularly as this population increases in size. Estimates are that as many as a half million older persons experience mistreatment annually in the UK (Action on Elder Abuse, 2005) and closer to two million cases of elder neglect and abuse occur each year in the US (National Research Council, 2003). Analysts acknowledge that elder mistreatment is more widespread than the known "cases" managed in health care settings and/or adult protective services; perhaps as few as one in five mistreated elders has been identified (National Center of Elder Abuse, 1998). Disturbingly, data from the UK show that as many as one-third of adults have never heard the term "elder abuse" (Help the Aged, 2006). But when probed, four-fifths of adults can identify an older adult man or woman who they think has been mistreated (Action on Elder Abuse). It is quite likely that similar levels of (un)familiarity occur in the US.

Even though people seem to "know" that elder mistreatment exists, there exists far less understanding of older men's experiences with abuse and neglect and what places older men at differential risk than older women. Questions about how many older men are neglected and/or abused and what makes older men vulnerable to mistreatment require gendered answers as well as a gendered framework for understanding men's later life vulnerabilities. However, with the exception of Kosberg (1998; Kosberg & Bowie, 1997), researchers interested in late life masculinities (e.g., Arber, Davidson, & Ginn, 2003; Thompson, 1994) often have not raised questions about older men's mistreatment, and few gerontologists who see late life through a "gendered lens" have questioned if men's old-age vulnerabilities are equivalent to women's (Mouton, Talamantes, Parker, Espino, & Miles, 2001). The basic problem with earlier analyses of elder mistreatment is the absence of a concern with gender (Whittaker, 1995), especially the way gendered policies and procedures yield men's mistreatment. This article begins with the premise that social processes do generate unequal exposure to risks, making older men (and women) differentially vulnerable.

THEORETICAL CONSIDERATION

The nation's knowledge of men's mistreatment is based largely on the cases reported to state protection agencies. However, older men who have encountered mistreatment are likely to not seek help from outsiders for a variety of reasons (cf., Addis & Mahalik, 2003; Brown, 2000; Sellers, Jackson, & Hardison, 1998), and gatekeepers to health and social services too frequently take no action to report men's mistreatment (cf., Dyer, Connolly, & McFeeley, 2003; Kennedy, 2005; Rodriguez, Wallace, Woolf, & Mangoine, 2006). Conventional wisdom proposes that women are more likely victimized in Western societies, and the expectation is that women will more likely report their experiences with abuse. In fact, with the one exception of abandonment, the majority of those who are known to suffer neglect and abuse are older women (National Research Council, 2003). Because the official statistics intuitively "make sense," few people question how the data are influenced by gender. But the power of gender ideologies to shape perceptions and expectations even in face of contrary evidence (Lorber, 1994), the acceptance of the feminization of victimization in our culture (Lisak, 1993), gendered assumptions about self-determination, and/or gatekeepers' lack of training in identifying men's experiences with abuse and neglect (Dyer, 2005; Kennedy) yield a type of pluralistic ignorance about older men's neglect and abuse.

As a social institution intertwined with the state and other institutions, gender matters (Connell, 1987; Martin, 2004). It influences what we know about elder mistreatment. Connell and Martin have urged people to recognize that gender structures social interaction, establishes expectations for individuals, orders social processes, and is built into the major social organizations of society. On one hand, men themselves may be less ready to talk about the physical abuse and neglect they experience, when they recognize it. No matter from what subculture old men originate, the masculinities they live by seem to be "collective" in at least one sense–men neither make much of the various forms of harassment and mistreatment they encounter, nor dwell on the painful incidents of mistreatment (Wood, 2006). The "tough guise" masculinity expectations persuade men to not interpret mistreatment as mistreatment, rather to normalize it. Even when men recognize their experiences as neglect and abuse, many are not likely to step forward and identify themselves as victims. Masculinity practices silence men, and their silence thwarts our understanding.

In Western cultures, men's experiences with mistreatment are also normalized by others. As part of the social organization of masculinity, and thus as ordinary *for men*, people have long normalized men's experiences with violence–whether it is the brutality of war witnessed by WWII veterans (Spiro, Schnurr, & Aldwin, 1994), being an ethnic Chinese-American and "not standing a Chinaman's chance" (Kingston, 1977), African American or Native American men's lifelong struggle for respect from the dominant culture (Duneier, 1992; Silko, 1997), or the traumatic injuries and violent crime associated with the men on America's social margins (Cohen, 1999; Dietz & Wright, 2005a). Without intending to, the images that people maintain of men normalize and naturalize older men's experiences with mistreatment. They are perceived by everyone around them as men, not just an elder (Hearn, 1995; Thompson, 2006). "Being a man" is an expectation that extends into late life, normalizing older men's mistreatment with the idioms "He can handle it, because he has been through worse" or "He's smart; he would know the difference."

In addition, gender is an underpinning for agency policies and procedures that affect whether or not an older man's mistreatment is identified as elder abuse and neglect. The double jeapordy of being an old man can produce discrimination and normalize mistreatment. When emergency room physicians send homeless men "home," when protective agency workers do not rescue an old man from the intentional neglect of a board-and-care facility because the old man is afraid of leaving his only "home," when the police view the misdemeanors and felonies that are linked to *domestic* violence as elder abuse but exclude the intentional neglect and financial abuse men more often experience, or when police officers interpret an old gay man's victimization as only a hate crime against sexuality, these actions can be interpreted as evidence of the sexism and ageism that mask the nation's understanding of the mistreatment experienced by populations of old men.

Ironically, mistreatment of elder men has been normalized for centuries: Older men's mistreatment is discussed in Ancient Greek mythology (e.g., Erinyes) and Shakespeare's depiction of the aged father's neglect and abuse by his daughters in *King Lear*. Even contemporary geriatric clinicians use the name of the stubborn, cynical, eccentric Greek philosopher Diogenes to describe a "syndrome" of so-called self-neglect (Payne & Gainey, 2005), which is gendered and descriptive of community-dwelling antisocial, self-reliant old men. Older men's neglect and abuse is certainly not ahistorical, nor does it occur in a vacuum. Many of the determinants of older men's mistreatment remain hidden, masked within cultural discourses and routine activities.

OLDER MEN'S VULNERABILITIES

Rather than concentrate on what individual characteristics put old men at risk, the authors investigated how gendered practices and social policies elevate the risks of older men's mistreatment. On one hand is the *de facto* sexism evident in institutional practices, such as the normative character of protocols for managing agitated men in nursing homes that call for pharmaceutical straight-jackets to keep in check their assertiveness (Burgio, Butler, Roth, Hardin, Hsu, & Ung, 2000; Schneider et al., 2006; Zun, 2003). There is also the accepted practice of gatekeepers' decisions to not report elder abuse when presented by older men (McCreadie, Bennett, Gilthorpe, Houghton, & Tinker, 2000). Additionally is the *de jure* sexism evident in social policy, such as hospital protocols for managing homeless men's hypothermia (Kruger & Moon, 1999) as "self-neglect" and not as evidence of the social neglect that causes the homelessness. Another example of *de jure* sexism is found in states where the adult's right to self-determination *permits* health care professionals and elder protective service workers to allow avidly self-reliant old men with mild cognitive and memory impairments to be left in (or returned to) an abusive home. Kahan and Paris (2003) detail a case of how Mr. R.'s well-documented history of physical abuse and neglect resulted in a thick case file but no successful rescue from the abusive son. The son's mistreatment also was not reported to protective services by the health care professionals. The "right" of the managed care plan to characterize the son's sickening neglect that caused the old man's wounds as beyond medical concern and the absence of someone challenging the older man's right to self-determination permitted the older man to be left in an abusive environment.

Whether it is "in principle" or "in practice," there are policies and practices that boost the likelihood that older men are at risk of mistreatment. Throughout this article, an ethnographic approach is used that draws on particulars, or cases, collected from news accounts, conversations with elder protective service investigators, and published research. From the particulars, the authors theorize that older men's probability of experiencing neglect and abuse is elevated by institutionalized practices and social policies.

Vulnerability to Abuse by Family and Trusted Others

One of the more damaging aspects of ageism is when older men internalize the message they learned as younger men: as old men they do not measure up anymore (cf., Levy, 2003; Thompson, 2006). For men in later life "a key issue is the maintenance of masculinity and autonomy" (Arber et al., 2003, p. 11), despite changes in their circumstances. Among the many elder mistreatment scenarios, one of the more disquieting ones is when older men are mistreated by their families. The current generation of older men has tried to live in sync with a construction of masculinity that expected men to strive for the "package deal"– employment, marriage, family, home ownership (Townsend, 2002). The mandate to provide a single-family home in a safe neighborhood with good schools and opportunities for children perpetuates the image of men as their family's providers and protectors. Gender ideologies also call for a man to resist being pushed around by others. It follows that when old men are neglected, abused, and exploited by family members or intimates, their sense of self can be emasculated–they recognize that they can no longer even protect themselves (personal communication, Elder Protective Services investigator). As well, the neglect and financial abuse they typically experience tend to be *felt* as a betrayal of trust rather than *perceived* as outright theft and abandonment (Wilber & Reynolds, 1996).

Being abused by a family member may be more troubling for old men than the abuse and neglect itself. Unable to embody masculinity, men can feel ashamed of what the mistreatment may imply about themselves *as men*, even when they know it was not possible or reasonable to defend themselves (cf., Barer, 1997). As Pritchard (2001, p. 57) observed in her UK study of older men's victimization, "All the men interviewed had a sense of resignation about what had happened to them, whether the abuse had been experienced in the past or very recently. None of them presented as embittered but rather with a sense of sadness."

Thus, in situations where the neglect and abuse are fully recognized by older men, they may feel there is little they can do. Their reasons not to seek help are varied. They may feel emasculated and ashamed, not want the abusing relative arrested, fear retaliation, genuinely believe they can manage the problem, and/or feel more harm might occur from reporting. The neglect and financial abuse they typically experience tend to be felt as a betrayal of trust rather than perceived as outright theft and abandonment (Wilber & Reynolds, 1996).

Beard and Payne's (2005) study of the reports of elder abuse in national newspapers found neglect cases were infrequently reported, even though neglect, improper use of medicines, and abandonment are the most common forms of old men's mistreatment. What the public often reads in newspaper accounts are the most egregious cases of financial abuse (Beard & Payne). On the rise and becoming the most prevalent type of mistreatment, the financial abuse that older men experience is typically involved with other forms of abuse, especially physical neglect (cf., Dimah & Dimah, 2002). Occurring more among the middle and working class, it can be as simple as the taking of money from an older man or as elaborate as coercing him into signing over real estate or other assets under false pretenses.

Financial abuse is more commonly perpetrated by adult children, and it is the fathers, not mothers, who are the usual target. In abusive families, older men are repositioned from active protectors and providers into silenced victims who often are expected to still provide. In one case, a frail 79-year-old man shared his home with a niece and nephew, who convinced him to pay them $1200 a month to live there. Verbally abusive, they guilted him when he mused about moving out. He was systematically isolated and became a prisoner in his own home (Caccamise, 2006).

Older men seem special "marks" because of their proclivity to not divulge a violation of a trusted relationship and because they tend to have more financial resources than older women. A case described on the American Psychological Association's (2005) online public interest directorate reveals one older man's vulnerability:

> James is a financially secure 90-year-old man who has been healthy and active until the last year. He has finally agreed to move in with

his oldest daughter . . . who now believes her father 'owes her' more of his money than her brother and two sisters are entitled to. She talks her father into giving her power of attorney . . . Soon she has come up with excuses to transfer a significant portion of his investment holdings into her name . . .

This is not an isolated case, and financial abuse may entail Kosberg's (1998) idea of "pay back," where an adult child who has been mistreated by the older man at some earlier point in their family history takes some revenge.

The National Elder Abuse Incidence Study (National Center on Elder Abuse, 1998) determined that 12 percent of all the reported and substantiated elder abuse cases were financial exploitation, whereas Wilber and Reynolds (1996) estimated that when undetected cases are taken into account, financial abuse may total one-half of all elder abuse in the United States. Among the abused men Pritchard (2001) identified, all were physically or emotionally isolated within their families. "Sam, who was kept in one room by his wife and daughter, was 'let out' only when he came to [the] day centre [once a week]; he did 'sneak out' once to seek advice from a solicitor about obtaining a divorce" (p. 83). The men became emasculated, home-bound prisoners while they continued to be providers; yet, because it is their family, only one-third made a conscious decision to leave their abusive environment. Whether it is the "silenced provider" or the "caregiver stress" hypothesis that explains older men's mistreatment in trusted relationships, men seem resigned to live with their situation, and some blame themselves. As an old Hispanic man, cited in Kahan and Paris (2003, p. 67) stated: "I am a burden to my son."

There is compelling evidence that these "silenced men" are more common than first thought. In one publicized case, an unreasonably confined man lived with his wife, who was his legal guardian. He was not allowed to see his siblings or grandchildren, and his wife constructed an eight-foot fence with blue tarps around the residence. Despite testimony by the Executive Director of the State Council on Elder Abuse and Neglect that the man's isolation was abusive, a probate court refused to redefine the husband-wife relationship and amend the guardianship. The man was denied the rights and privileges the State of Georgia guarantees as a convicted criminal (Twitty, 1999). Similarly, Sacks (2001) details a case where an older man's trailer home was burglarized and his possessions stolen or vandalized by his vindictive ex-wife. The man felt trapped, a prisoner of his ex-wife's harassment, and he worried about the criminal justice system's propensity to stand ready to jail him on the accusation of the woman who victimized him: "If I call the police, she'll say I attacked her . . . If I try to defend my home and come near her, she'll scream, call the police and I'll go to jail." Whether this older man's worried beliefs are valid or not, the case helps illustrate some men's perception of the gendered practices within social institutions that "ratchet down" the prospect of the men protecting themselves. Understanding men's perceptions of the sexism they perceive in policies and practices might well help us understand their help seeking (or lack there of).

Unless it is a case of flagrant abuse, men's mistreatment is not apt to capture public attention (cf., Beard & Payne, 2005). In practice, the doctrine of family privacy suggests that what goes on inside family households generally stays inside the family (Berardo, 1998). In principle, the concept of *la familia*, where the honor of the family is perceived as greater than the needs of the individual (Montoya, 1997), is not restricted to Spanish-speaking communities but is a more universal dimension of masculinity in American culture. The importance ascribed to the family and family privacy in custom and in law allows harmful behavior to go unnoticed and unreported, even for older men. Add adults' right to self-determination and the US legal system assures the principles that privacy and autonomy can be more important than older men's safety.

Because the doctrine of family privacy quietly allows an old man to "choose" to live in harm's way, provided he is competent to choose, old men often do choose to not seek-help. They try to tough it out. Disturbingly, the trauma arising from men's experience of mistreatment goes unnoticed. Reel (1997, p. 107) suggests that physical or emotional neglect yields passive trauma. "Rather than a violence presence, passive trauma may be defined as a violent lack–the absence of nurture and [care work] normally expected of a caregiver." When untreated, passive trauma becomes a basis for depression (Reel) and suicidal tendencies, especially among men who hold traditional views of masculinity (Hinton, Zweifach, Oishi, Tang, & Unützer, 2006). In the US, men accounted for 82 percent of the suicides among older adults (Centers for Disease Control and Prevention, 1999). Older men living with mistreatment are also at a higher risk for unhealthy coping mechanisms (e.g., alcohol/substance use) and re-victimization. By comparison, the trauma arising from a family member's verbal and physical abuse is "a clearly toxic interaction" (Reel, p. 107), and it is injurious. Bachman, Lachs, and Meloy (2004) reported that nearly three-fourths of older men injured by family members required medical care for their injuries, compared to one-half of older women.

Older gays also may end up "self-neglecting" in order to protect themselves from others' homophobia, since help-seeking might require outing oneself (Cook-Daniels, 1997). Cook-Daniels noted that older gays tend to refuse home care services, fearing that a worker might become abusive or blackmail them because of their sexuality, and they refuse to move into senior housing because they have nothing in common with their heterosexual peers. Similarly, Hispanics' and African Americans' wariness of the criminal justice system and skepticism of outsiders (Brown, 2000; Duneier, 1992; Montoya, 1997; Sellers, Jackson, & Hardison, 1998) makes its difficult for abused older men to reveal their mistreatment.

Vulnerability to Nursing Home/Institutional Abuse

Although there has been little attention paid to the gendered nature of elder mistreatment in residential care settings (Aitken & Griffin 1996), it can be argued that older men living in institutional and congregate settings are particularly vulnerable to neglect and abuse. Nursing homes are distinctly gendered. The feminization of residential care settings is rooted in sex-ratios: The majority of nursing home residents are women, and the vast majority of paid carers are women; thus, older men in most residential settings live in a markedly female environment (cf., Paoletti, 2002). Review a monthly activities calendar for a typical nursing home in Massachusetts, and perhaps one event sticks out as being attractive to men–a bi-weekly one-hour men's breakfast. The remainder of the planned activities for the residents–from the films shown to the music and movement type activities–are not consonant with men's interests *as men*. Ironically, older men are more inclined to use therapeutic recreational services than the women (McDonald, Nyankori, & McGuire, 1996). In the end, older men living in most residential care facilities are obliged to participate in demasculinzing activities if they seek any social involvement.

The intended practices of residential care facilities are to recognize the uniqueness of each resident, but intentions give way to the day-to-day practices of the underpaid, largely female staff that, by necessity, ritualizes care work. Often homogenized into child-like "residents," the unique needs of men become superfluous to the day-to-day operation of the residential facilities (Caporael, 1981; Diamond, 1995). "The removal of decision-making powers, the lack of privacy and the infantilization experienced in institutions all contribute to [institutional mistreatment]" (Aitken & Griffin, 1996, p. 85). But it is more than staffing issues that undermine older men's sense of themselves as men. A 67-year-old journalist, who was a patient in the rehabilitative wing of a nursing home, commented:

> The diminutives! The endearments! The idiotic *we*'s. Hello, dear, how are we today? What's your name, dear? Shall we go to the dining room? Hi, hon, sorry to take so long. Don't we look nice today! You've got to eat, sweetie. Sweetie, would you take a pill for me? A little prune juice, sweetie? Chirpy singsong voices. Who thinks we want to be talked to this way? (Corbet, 2007)

Residents' experience of passive and intentional neglect far exceeds their experience of abuse (Hawes, 2003; MacDonald, 2000); yet, abuse occurs. Should men become agitated as a result of their dismissed masculinity and/or enforced isolation, it is likely that their agitation will be controlled with chemical or increased physical restraints (Burgio et al., 2000), and this resistance-control tug-of-war between the man and the staff can spiral down and result in less meaningful interaction with staff (Allen, Burgio, Fisher, Hardin, & Shuster, 2005).

A survey of nurses and nurse aides who were employed in 31 different nursing homes in New Hampshire found that 36 percent of the nursing and aide staff reported having witnessed at least one incident of physical abuse by other staff members in the preceding year. Ten percent admitted to committing at least one act of physical abuse themselves (Pillemer & Moore, 1989). Psychological abuse–yelling at a resident, insulting or swearing at a resident–was observed by 81 percent of the staff, and 40 percent admitted to committing such an act (Pillemer & Moore). In two other studies (MacDonald, 2000; Pillemer & Hudson, 1993) of nursing home staff who participated in abuse-prevention training, more than half admitted to having yelled, insulted, or swore at a resident and nearly one-tenth divulged that they had been physically aggressive.

One of the key predictors of staff-initiated physical and psychological abuse on nursing home residents is a staff member's prior experience with residents' physical aggressiveness (Pillemer & Bachman-Prehn, 1991). Is mistreatment of men in institutional settings simply *quid pro quo*? No, the mistreatment old men face is structurally rooted in staff's gendered practices as much as their poor training and insufficient supervision. The physical aggression by staff has been accounted for as a type of accepted reflective-action and self-protection, as exemplified by a nurse aide's comment: "If I grab him and sit him down, or even shove him into his chair to keep him from biting me, [that] is not abuse. . . . If I'm rough with him, I'm just protecting myself from injury" (cited in Hawes, 2003, p. 485). In the dominant culture, men are routinely *perceived* as more violent than women, even though incidents of violence by long-term residents toward the residential care workers rarely affirm this sex-difference (cf., Burgio et al., 2000). Although their study is not a direct parallel, Bachman, Lachs, and Meloy (2004, pp. 20-21) reported that "physical resistance appears to have a price in attacks perpetrated by known offenders . . . men's fighting back esculated the level of violence experienced."

The mistreatment of men goes beyond the gendered practices of poorly trained, overworked staff who perceive men as potentially violent and normalize their *quid pro quo* neglect and abuse (Payne, Berg, & James, 2001). Mistreatment occurs in a context where there is the absence of vigilant ombudsmen and the timely enforcement of "mandatory" reporting. The law in some states "urges" but does not require professionals and others who are in a position to detect mistreatment to report it. Perhaps more telling, the problem of timely enforcement is exemplified by the year and half between when a certified nursing assistant (CNA) was criminally charged for twice tripping a 74-year-old man and striking him on the head and tormenting a 76-year-old partially deaf man by repeatedly striking the man in his hearing aid (Office of the Massachusetts Attorney General, 2006). In the interim between his dismissal from the nursing home and his arrest, the abusive CNA worked the 18 months in another nursing home. In another case, a trained investigator in New Mexico assumed the undercover role of an Alzheimer's resident in a lockdown unit where, because of staffing shortages, he was neglected: "I never took a shower or changed my clothes the entire [five days] I was there" (Basler, 2004). He was "allowed" to be self-sufficient. Whether these cases illustrate only the quality of care of badly run residential facilities or the systemic failure to perceive men's neglect and abuse as gendered mistreatment has never been investigated.

Despite contested estimates that suggest older men's mistreatment is more prevalent in institutional settings than family settings (Hawes, 2003; Pillemer & Finkelhor, 1988), it is ironic that the Pillemer and Bachman-Prehn (1991) study is the only one the authors found that tried to account for what determined nursing home staffs' mistreatment of an older adult. No study has determined if older men are vulnerable because of their masculinity performances, as has been suggested. It is the absence of research that provokes the question: what makes older men who live in nursing homes, adult congregate housing, and board-and-care facilities particularly vulnerable to staff mistreatment–to rough handling, pinching, pushing, slapping and hitting, swearing, or decisions to intentionally skip the body work needed for basic hygiene? Clearly, the older men (and women) who live in long-term care settings are vulnerable by definition, and many require help with dressing, bathing, and other activities of daily living (Hawes, 2003). But frailty and dependency are *not* directly associated with abuse (Reis & Nahmiash, 1999). So, what determines institutionalized older men's mistreatment? It is believed that gender ideologies and practices are significant.

Hawes (2003) proposed that dependency may make men feel it necessary to silently endure physical and chemical restraints, personal attacks, and neglect. But is being silent characteristic of *most* old men living in institutional settings? It is thought not, and argued here that older men are more likely to continue to engage in masculinity performances and resist, or act out against, the expectations to be a passive resident; they refuse to forego "being a man." Gerschick and Miller (1994) observed that men with health disabilities often continue to take control of their own lives, and "their sense of control is more than mere illusion" (p. 38). Men reformulate their masculinity performances to fit their limitations. It is not surprising that even when bedridden, men continue to embody masculinity and draw on a gender-based set of interaction strategies. They see themselves reflected in their actions. In Tracey Kidder's *Old Friends* (1994), one of the two old men, Joe, is a curmudgeon whose gender repertoire affirmed his desire to control his body and time (and regularly watch his Red Soxs). Joe could have been intentionally neglected and/or garnered rough handling in a different residential care facility. Men in a state of confinement, their freedom drastically curtailed by their health status and/or staff's use of physical and chemical restraints, may seek alternative means to feel "in control." As they renounce institutional efforts to demasculinize them, their verbal and behavioral insistence to be treated respectfully as a man could provoke "pay back" abuse and neglect (Kosberg & Bowie, 1997) from the staff that literally and figuratively put older men "in their place."

It is theorized that the neglect men experience is as much a gendered response to being an older man as it is evidence of systemic organizational problems. The *de facto* sexism of using pharmaceutical restraints to manage men's frustrations, and the perceived legitimacy of staff members' rough handling of men's noncompliant attitude and behaviors, suggest that men may well be at greater risk of elder mistreatment because of the gendered practices of care workers and the policies within residential care facilities that demasculinize the men.

Vulnerability to Public Abuse and Neglect

There are many public policies and traditions that jeopardize some populations of old men more than others. The purpose of this section is to illustrate the way gendered practices and policies differentially affect populations of older men. Of necessity, this section is selective and omits worthy research and policy issues.

Older men are often victimized in the community. Especially vulnerable are men who maintain high-risk lifestyles, who live alone, are near-homeless or live on the streets, drink heavily, and/or have insufficient financial means. These are the men who are misdiagnosed as "self-neglecting," when in fact they are neglected by the nation and are more likely to die prematurely (Lachs, Williams, O'Brien, Pillemer, & Charlson, 1998). The use of the construct "self-neglecting" sanitizes the mistreatment that is done to the men and essentializes the injuries of mistreatment as originating in individual pathology. When a socially marginal man seeks medical care for several large venous ulcers, but his protein-energy malnutrition, wasting, dementia-like symptoms, and depression are not his part of presenting complaint, the etiology of this man's presenting problems often will be defined as "self-neglect" (Abrams, Lachs, McAvay, Keohane, & Bruce, 2002; Pavlou & Lachs, 2006). His chronic medical needs can go untreated.

Recognizing the complexity of the needs of neglected and abused men, Callahan (1988) has argued against specialized protective service intervention and for a national effort to remove marginalized men from society's margins: "[The] greatest abuse that can beset older persons [is the] failure to provide them with the economic means for a decent life and opportunities to exercise their own choices" (p. 458). The authors agree. Most of the time older men's mistreatment cannot be interpreted with ungendered, individualistic models of risk (Sprey & Matthews, 1989), nor can such adversities be remedied through "Band-Aids" administered "downstream" that try to rescue already victimized individuals. There is a need to "look upstream" (McKinlay, 1979) to the structural and societal neglect, and the underlying disrespectful and ageist attitudes, that disfavor older men.

The financial exploitation of older men by people outside their families is an illustrative case. Prevention does not address the systemic problems; rather, it is individualized through mass media reports of uncommon cases or suggestions for "education" campaigns (Wolf & Pillemer, 1994). A news report of two elder women's alleged hit-and-run murders exemplifies older, socially marginal men being preyed upon: "According to the authorities, the two women extended help to two homeless men, getting them off the streets and putting them up in apartments, while at the same time plotting their deaths. Posing as aunts, fiancées or cousins, they took out numerous life insurance policies on the men . . . with themselves as the beneficiaries" (Chang, 2006, p. A12). The women had befriended vulnerable men, were profiting from them, and used the insurance industry to extract more than $2 million from insurance policies. This pair of "cases" educates indirectly; it reveals the way gendered policies within the insurance industry, health and social services agencies, pension plans, police protocols, and many other domains put older men at risk of mistreatment.

The irony is that despite the extent of financial abuse that occurs, fewer than ten states mandate that professionals in the financial field report suspected abuse. The abuse remains invisible. A lack of case law on elder abuse also seriously compounds the problem for officers of the court seeking legal recourse for crimes against older men. But as Callahan (1988) and McKinlay (1979) cautioned, such downstream interventions may rescue some of those in need but do not address the social problem. Hodge's (2006) testimony to the White House Conference Aging draws attention to the need for regulatory protection:

> As we have seen with what is happening to the US Pension Benefit Guaranty Corporation, . . . we have witnessed tens of thousands of private pensions/401K's being wiped out and/or severely depleted because of poor corporate governance practices and/or corporate accounting shenanigans, greed, corruption and 'old fashioned' criminal behavior . . . The consequences of these crimes and poor corporate governance practices have a far greater impact and more lasting effect on an aging victim's life than on a younger adult's. Being swindled out of your life savings and supplemental retirement income by a stock/accounting fraud scam may be an extremely negative experience for a thirty year old but it is absolutely devastating and, indeed, life threatening to a seventy-six year-old trying to make ends meet with just Social Security payments and no prospect of earning the stolen money back.

Unlike the UK and Canadian societies, social policy in the US positions many men to be at risk of mistreatment in later life. Employment is the core dimension of the "package deal" that defines manhood and respectability (Duneier, 1992; Townsend, 2001), and employment status is linked to health care. Consequently, the men who were always marginally employed (cf., Gibson, 1993) and the long-term unemployed old men cannot afford to purchase medical services within American private-pay health care system, and many proudly abstain from asking for complimentary help from emergency departments until their conditions are grave. Some of the men are forced to choose between food, housing, and medical services. From the outside looking in, it may appear that a socially-marginal older man is choosing to self-neglect when in fact he simply cannot afford to adequately provide for all his needs.

Are these patterns of systemic neglect sufficiently gendered to make old men more at risk than old women? Regardless of reports that older men and women are equally vulnerable to physical assault (cf., Dietz and Wright, 2005b), earlier investigations are overpopulated with poor, older women who have "homes" and underrepresented by the men in the urban underclass. Not recognized are the "Veteran fraternities" of near-homeless and homeless men whose war-related stressors, social isolation, and substance abuse are correlated with physical violence and traumatic injuries. Wright and Weber (1987) reported that traumatic injury is among the top presenting complaints to emergency medical services. Also not recognized are the "rough sleepers" who are almost exclusively men, at risk to the extremes of violence, and totaled 18,384 emergency room visits in Boston hospitals in a four-year period (O'Connell, Roncarati, Reilly et al., 2004). This population is clearly at risk of traumatic injury. Disturbingly, Messman (2005) details the emergence of six "Bumfights" videos where homeless old men are dehumanized as targets for physical assaults and beatings by young men engaged in their own masculinity performances.

CLOSING THOUGHTS

The estimates of older men's mistreatment and the underlying true prevalence of their experiences with mistreatment have been described metaphorically as the "tip of the iceberg" (Cyphers, 1999; National Center of Elder Abuse, 1998). When data-gathering shifts away from using state protection agencies' reported cases and toward population-based surveys, the estimate of older men's victimization is more alarming. Pillemer and Finkelhor (1988) discovered the per capita rate of victimization for men was nearly double that for women–5.1% of older men versus 2.5% of older women. Their findings were (and are) perplexing, given the prevailing gender expectation that presumes men would not as often be victims. They tried to explain their findings in terms of a sex-difference in living arrangements: Shared residence increases men's risk. Perhaps, however, men's lifetime experiences with various forms of aggression influence their own perceptions and interpretations of vulnerability. When men participate in a population survey, such as undertaken by Pillemer and Finkelhor (1988) or Comijs, Pot, Smit, Bouter, and Jonker (1998), in which they were asked to divulge their *everyday* experiences, they can matter-of-factly disclose an abusive experience without personally labeling their experience as "victimization." The men can talk about being hit, scratched, or having to routinely live with denigrating verbal assaults without help-seeking, initiating a protective services report, or interpreting their experiences in an unmanly "I am (and allowed myself to become) a victim." Very likely, many men in the Boston sample normalized their mistreatment, much as caregiving husbands accept their wives' physical aggression (Calasanti, 2006).

Older men's mistreatment is normalized in many other ways. The gender ideologies guiding people's understanding of older men commonly lead to the perception of men as self-sufficient and self-reliant. It is thus not surprising that a good proportion of the mistreatment encountered by the urban underclass, which is overrepresented by men, is normalized as "self-neglect." Defining societal neglect (Callahan, 1988) as self-neglect, or interpreting the intentional neglect of informal and paid caregivers in terms of "he can handle it," results in fewer trauma-based services available to men. Many elder abuse support groups, shelters, and programs serve only female victims.

Existing roadblocks to understanding older men's mistreatment and thus prevention fall into several categories. First is the hesitancy of victims to reach out and engage services, as was noted above. Also noted above, mandated professionals and front-line practitioners become barriers when they are unclear as to what constitutes men's mistreatment, lack knowledge about appropriate resources for older men, or simply are unwilling to intervene (Rodriguez et al., 2006). The most significant is a societal level roadblock, as evidenced by the near absence of preventive efforts for this social problem and, by comparison, the dominance of a "downstream" rescue approach to interventions and the funding of services. What is missing in nearly all public reports and services is explicit recognition of how gender matters. Power issues are as central to men's mistreatment in later life as women's. Older men's financial exploitation by relatives (as well as the physical abuse, abandonment, and neglect that many older men live with at home, in institutions, and on the street) hinges on power inequalities. It is time for gerontologists and gender scholars to step back and assess the "upstream" determinants of men's risks for elder abuse and neglect. No adequate theory or intervention can be developed unless the gender issues inherent in men's mistreatment are recognized to be a product of complex gendered practices and policies.

REFERENCES

Abrams, R. C., Lachs, M., McAvay, G., Keohane, D. J., & Bruce, M. J. (2002). Predictors of self-neglect in community-dwelling elders. *American Journal of Psychiatry, 159*, 1724-1730.

Action on Elder Abuse. (2005). *Hidden voices: Older people's experiences of abuse.* London: Astral House.

Addis, M. E, & Mahalik, J. R. (2003). Men, masculinity, and the contexts of help seeking. *American Psychologist, 58*, 5-14.

Aitken, L., & Griffin, G. (1996). *Gender issues in elder abuse.* London: Sage Publications.

Allen, R. S., Burgio, L. D., Fisher, S. E., Hardin, J. M., & Shuster, J. L. (2005). Behavioral characteristics of agitated nursing home residents with dementia at the end of life. *The Gerontologist, 45*, 661-666.

American Psychological Association. (2005). *Aging issues: Elder abuse and neglect: In search of solutions.* Washington, DC.: American Psychological Association. Retrieved August 30, 2006 from http://www.apa.org/pi/aging/eldabuse.html

Arber, S., Davidson, K., & Ginn, J. (2003). *Gender and ageing: Changing roles and relationships.* Maidenhead, England: Open University Press.

Bachman, R., Lachs, M., & Meloy, M. (2004). Reducing injury through self-protection by elderly victims of violence: The interaction effects of gender of victim and the victim/offender relationship. *Journal of Elder Abuse & Neglect, 16*(4), 1-24.

Barer, B. M. (1997). The secret shame of the very old: "I've never told this to anyone else." *Journal of Mental Health and Aging, 3*, 365-375.

Basler, B. (2004, September). Undercover resident: The nursing home staff thought he was failing. Turns out they were. *AARP Bulletin.* Retrieved October 29, 2006 from http://www.aarp.org/bulletin/yourhealth/Articles/a2004-08-26-undercover. html

Beard, H., & Payne, B. K. (2005). The portrayal of elder abuse in the national media. *American Journal of Criminal Justice, 29*, 269-284.

Berardo, F. M. (1998). Family privacy: Issues and concepts. *Journal of Family Issues, 19*, 4-19.

Brown, E. A. (2000). Elder mistreatment in the African American community. *African American Research Perspectives, 6,* 105-114.

Burgio, L. D., Butler, F. R., Roth, D. L., Hardin, J. M., Hsu, C., & Ung, K. (2000). Agitation in nursing home residents: The role of gender and social context. *International Psychogeriatrics, 12,* 495-511.

Caccamise, P. L. (2006, June 15). Help elders who are victims of abuse, neglect, exploitation. *Rochester Democrat and Chronicle.* Retrieved August 29, 2006 from http://www.democratandchronicle.com/

Calasanti, T. M. (2006). Gender and old age: Lessons from spousal care work. In T. Calasanti & K. F. Slevin (Eds.), *Age matters: Realigning feminist thinking* (pp. 269-294). New York: Routledge.

Callahan, J. (1988). Elder abuse: Some questions for policy-makers. *The Gerontologist, 28,* 453-458.

Caporael, L. R. (1981). The paralanguage of caregiving: Baby talk to the institutionalized aged. *Journal of Personality and Social Psychology, 40,* 876-884.

Centers for Disease Control and Prevention. (1999, December 17). Surveillance for selected public health indicators affecting older adults–United States. *MMWR, 48* (No. SS-8).

Chang, S. (2006, June 12). Two elderly women suspected as femmes fatales in insurance scheme fraud. *New York Times,* p. A12.

Cohen, C, I. (1999). Aging and homelessness. *The Gerontologist, 39,* 5-14.

Comijs, H. C., Pot, A. M., Smit, J. H., Bouter, L. M., & Jonker, C. (1998). Elder abuse in the community: Prevalence and consequences. *Journal of the American Geriatrics Society, 46,* 885-998.

Connell, R. W. (1987). *Gender and power.* Palo Alto: Stanford University Press.

Cook-Daniels, L. (1997). Lesbian, gay male, bisexual and transgendered elders: Elder abuse and neglect issues. *Journal of Elder Abuse & Neglect, 9*(2), 35-49.

Corbet, B. (2007, January/February). Embedded: A no-holds barred report from inside a nursing home. *AARP magazine.* Retrieved December 2, 2006 from http://www.aarpmagazine.org/health/embedded.html

Cyphers, G. (1999). *Estimating elder abuse through community sentinels: Results of the National Elder Abuse Incidence Study.* Washington, DC: American Public Human Services Association.

Diamond, T. (1995). *Making gray gold.* Chicago: University of Chicago Press.

Dietz, T., & Wright J. D. (2005a). Victimization of the elderly homeless. *Care Management Journals, 6*(1), 15-21.

Dietz, T., & Wright J. D. (2005b). Age and gender differences and predictors of victimization of the older homeless. *Journal of Elder Abuse & Neglect, 17*(1), 37-60.

Dimah, A., & Dimah, K. P. (2002). Gender differences among abused older African Americans and African American abusers in an elder abuse provider agency. *Journal of Black Studies, 32,* 557-573.

Duneier, M. (1992). *Slim's table: Race, respectability, and masculinity.* Chicago: University of Chicago Press.

Dyer, C. B. (2005). Neglect assessment in elderly persons. *Journal of Gerontology: Medical Sciences, 60,* 1000-1001.

Dyer, C. B., Connolly, M., & McFeeley, P. (2003). The clinical and medical forensics of elder abuse and neglect. In National Research Council, *Elder mistreatment: Abuse, neglect, and exploitation in an aging America* (pp. 339-381). Washington, DC: National Academic Press.

Gerschick, T. J., & Miller, A. S. (1994). Coming to terms: Masculinity and physical disability. *Masculinities, 2*, 34-55.

Gibson, R. C. (1993). The black American retirement experience. In J. S. Jackson, L. M. Chatters, and R. J. Taylor (Eds.), *Aging in black America* (pp. 277-297). Thousand Oaks, CA: Sage Publications.

Hawes, C. (2003). Elder abuse in residential long-term care settings: What is known and what information is needed? In National Research Council, *Elder mistreatment: Abuse, neglect, and exploitation in an aging America* (pp. 466-500). Washington, DC: National Academic Press.

Hearn, J. (1995). Imaging the aging of men. In M. Featherstone & A. Wernick (Eds.), *Images of aging: Cultural representations of later life* (pp. 97-115). London: Routledge.

Help the Aged. (2006). *Elder abuse facts.* London: Help the Aged. Retrieved August 30, 2006 from http://www.iwill.co.uk/facts.aspx

Hinton, H., Zweifach, M., Oishi, S., Tang, L., & Unützer, J. (2006). Gender disparities in the treatment of late-life depression: Qualitative and quantitative findings from the IMPACT trial. *American Journal of Geriatric Psychiatry, 14*, 884-892.

Hodge, P. (2006). Living younger longer: Baby boomer challenges. *White House Conference on Aging: Final report to the President and the Congress.* Washington, DC. Retrieved October 14, 2006 from http://www.genpolicy.com/articles/2005_WHCoA_Policy_Committee_cv.html

Johnson, T. F. (1991). *Elder mistreatment: Deciding who is at risk.* New York: Greenwood Press.

Kahan, F. S., & Paris, B. E. C. (2003). Why elder abuse continues to elude the health care system. *The Mount Sinai Journal of Medicine, 70*, 62-68.

Kennedy, R. D. (2005). Elder abuse and neglect: The experience, knowledge, and attitudes of primary care physicians. *Family Medicine, 37*, 481-485.

Kidder, T. (1994). *Old friends.* New York: Houghton Mifflin.

Kingston, M. H. (1977). *China men.* New York: Alfred Knoff.

Kosberg, J. I. (1998). The abuse of elderly men. *Journal of Elder Abuse & Neglect, 9*(3), 69-88.

Kosberg, J. I., & Bowie, S. L. (1997). The victimization of elderly men. In J. I. Kosberg & L. W. Kaye (Eds.), *Elderly men: Special problems and professional challenges* (pp. 216-229). New York: Springer Publications.

Kruger, R. M., & Moon, C. H. (1999). Can you spot the signs of elder mistreatment? *Postgraduate Medicine, 166*, 169-183.

Lachs, M. S., Williams, C. S., O'Brien, S., Pillemer, K. A., & Charlson, M. E. (1998). The mortality of elder mistreatment. *Journal of the American Medical Association. 280*, 428-432.

Levy, B. R. (2003). Mind matters: Cognitive and physical effects of aging self-stereotypes. *Journals of Gerontology: Psychological Sciences, 58*, P203-P211.

Lisak, D. (1993). Men as victims: Challenging cultural myths. *Journal of Traumatic Stress, 6*, 577-580.

Lorber, J. (1994). *The paradoxes of gender.* New Haven: Yale University Press.

MacDonald, P. (2000). *Make a difference: Abuse/neglect pilot project.* Washington, DC: National Long-Term Care Ombudsman Resource Center.

Martin, P. Y. (2004). Gender as a social institution. *Social Forces, 82*, 1249-1273.

McCreadie, C., Bennett, G., Gilthorpe, M. S., Houghton, G., & Tinker, A. (2000). Elder abuse: Do general practitioners know or care? *Journal of the Royal Society of Medicine, 93*(2), 67-71.

McDonald, J. M., Nyankori, J., & McGuire, F. A. (1996). Therapeutic recreation in nursing home utilization: Probability estimates by gender. *Activities, Adaptation, & Aging, 32*(2), 1-20.

McKinlay, J. (1979). A case for refocusing upstream: The political economy of illness. In J. Gartley (Ed.), *Patients, physicians and illness: A sourcebook in behavioral science and health* (pp. 9-25). New York: Free Press.

Messman, T. (2005, September). The increase in hate crimes and homeless murders is a warning sign. *Street Spirit.* Oakland: American Friends Service Committee. Retrieved September 30, 2006 from http://www.thestreetspirit.org/September2005/murders.htm

Montoya, V. (1997). Understanding and combating elder abuse in Hispanic communities. *Journal of Elder Abuse & Neglect, 9*(2), 5-17.

Mouton, C. P., Talamantes, M., Parker, R. W., Espino, D. V., & Miles, T. P. (2001). Abuse and neglect in older men. *Clinical Gerontologist, 24*(3/4), 15-26.

National Center of Elder Abuse. (1998). *National elder abuse incidence survey: Final report.* Washington, DC: Administration on Aging.

National Research Council. (2003). *Elder mistreatment: Abuse, neglect and exploitation in an aging America.* R. J. Bonnie & R. B. Wallace (Eds.). Washington, DC: National Academic Press.

O'Connell, J. J., Roncarati, J. S., Reilly, E. C., Kane, C. A., Morrison, S. K., Swain, S. E. et al. (2004). Old and sleeping rough: Elderly homeless persons on the streets of Boston. *Care Management Journals, 5*, 101-106.

Office of the Massachusetts Attorney General. (2006, April 8). Nursing assistant sentenced to House of Correction for patient abuse of elder at Cape nursing home. Retrieved August 30, 2006 from http://www.ago.state.ma.us/sp.cfm?pageid=986&id=1399

Paoletti, I. (2002). Caring for older people: A gendered practice. *Discourse & Society, 13*, 805-817.

Pavlou, M. P., & Lachs, M. S. (2006). Could self-neglect in older adults be a geriatric syndrome? *Journal of the American Geriatrics Society, 54*, 831-842.

Payne, B. K., & Gainey, R. R. (2005). Differentiating self-neglect as a type of elder mistreatment: How do these cases compare to traditional types of elder mistreatment? *Journal of Elder Abuse & Neglect, 17*(1), 21-36.

Payne, B. K., Berg, B. L., & James, L. F. (2001). Attitudes about sanctioning elder abuse offenders among police chiefs, nursing home employees, and students. *International Journal of Offender Therapy and Comparative Criminology, 45*, 363-382.

Pillemer, K., & Bachman-Prehn, R. (1991). Helping and hurting: Predictors of mal-treatment of patients in nursing homes. *Research on Aging, 13*, 74-95.

Pillemer, K., & Finkelhor, D. (1988). The prevalence of elder abuse: A random sample survey. *The Gerontologist, 28*, 51-57.

Pillemer, K., & Hudson, B. (1993). A model abuse prevention program for nursing assistants. *The Gerontologist, 33*, 128-131.

Pillemer, K. & Moore, D. W. (1989). Abuse of patients in nursing homes: Findings from a survey of staff. *The Gerontologist, 29*, 314-320.

Pritchard, J. (2001). *Male victims of elder abuse: Their experience and needs.* London: Jessica Kingsley Publishers.

Reel, T. (1997). *I don't want to talk about it: Overcoming the secret legacy of male depression.* New York: Fireside.

Reis, M., & Nahmiash, D. (1998). Validation of the indicators of abuse (IOA) screen. *The Gerontologist, 38*, 471-480.

Rodriguez, M. A., Wallace, S. P., Woolf, N. H., & Mangoine, C. M. (2006). Mandatory reporting of elder abuse: Between a rock and a hard place. *Annuals of Family Medicine, 4*, 403-409.

Sacks, G. (2001, September 29). Prisoners in their own homes: Male victims of elder abuse. *Santa Clarita Signal.* Retrieved October 14, 2006 from http://www.glennjsacks.com/

Schneider, L., Tariot, P., Dagerman, K., Davis, S., Hsiao, J., Ismail, M. S. et al. (2006). Effectiveness of atypical antipsychotic drugs in patients with Alzheimer's disease. *New England Journal of Medicine, 355*, 1525-38.

Sellers, S. L., Jackson, J. S., & Hardison, C. (1998). Minority issues. In M. Hersen & V. Van Hasselt (Eds.), *Handbook of clinical geropsychology* (pp. 505-522). NY: Plenum.

Silko, L. M. (1977). *Ceremony.* New York: Penguin Books.

Spiro, A., Schnurr, P. P., & Aldwin, C. M. (1996). Combat-related posttraumatic stress disorder symptoms in older men. *Psychology and Aging, 9*, 17-26.

Sprey, J., & Matthews, S. H. (1989). The perils of drawing policy implications from research: The case of elder mistreatment. In R. Filinson & S. R. Ingman (Eds.), *Elder abuse: Practice and policy.* (pp. 51-61). New York: Human Sciences Press.

Thompson, E. H. (1994). *Older men's lives.* Thousand Oaks, CA: Sage Publications.

Thompson, E. H. (2006). Images of old men's masculinity: Still a man? *Sex Roles, 55*, 633-648.

Townsend, N. (2002). *The package deal: Marriage, work and fatherhood in men's lives.* Philadelphia PA: Temple University Press.

Twitty, J. L. (1999). Commentary: Some older people do not have the same rights as convicted criminals: Bill's story. *Journal of Ethics, Law, and Aging, 5*, 51-52.

Whittaker, T. (1995). Gender and elder abuse. In S. Arber, & J. Ginn, (Eds.), *Connecting gender & ageing: A sociological approach* (pp. 144-157). Buckingham, England: Open University Press.

Wilber, K., & Reynolds S. (1996). Introducing a framework for defining financial abuse of the elderly. *Journal of Elder Abuse & Neglect;* 8(2), 61-80.

Wolf, R. S. (2000). The nature and scope of elder abuse. *Generations, 24*(2), 6-13.

Wolf, R. S., & Pillemer, K. (1994). What's new in elder abuse programming? Four bright ideas. *The Gerontologist, 34,* 126-129.

Wood, J. T. (2006). *Gendered lives* (7th edition). Belmont, CA: Wadsworth Publishing Company.

Wright, J. D., & Weber, E. (1987). *Homelessness and health.* Washington, DC: McGraw-Hill.

Zun, L. S. (2003). A prospective study of the complication rate of use of patient restraint in the emergency department. *Journal of Emergency Medicine, 24,* 119-124.

doi:10.1300/J084v19n01_09

Intervention with Abused Older Males:
Conceptual and Clinical Perspectives

Lenard W. Kaye, DSW, PhD
Diane Kay, MSW
Jennifer A. Crittenden, MSW

SUMMARY. Men and women experience abuse in different ways and older men have particular treatment needs that must be addressed by clinicians. The current design and configuration of clinical services may create barriers to abused older men receiving treatment fully suited to their needs. In this article, the unique experiential dynamics and help seeking behaviors of older men who experience abuse are delineated and recommendations are given for structuring services to better meet their needs. Gender-sensitive clinical techniques and modalities are described and suggestions for interventions that could prove particularly efficacious in the treatment of older men are offered. doi:10.1300/J084v19n01_10 *[Article copies available for a fee from The Haworth Document Delivery Service: 1-800-HAWORTH. E-mail address: <docdelivery@haworthpress.com> Website: <http://www.HaworthPress.com> © 2007 by The Haworth Press, Inc. All rights reserved.]*

KEYWORDS. Older men, abuse, trauma, clinical treatment

Lenard W. Kaye is Professor at the University of Maine and Director of its Center on Aging (E-mail: Len.kaye@umit.main.edu). Diane Kay is a Graduate Assistant (E-mail: Diane.kay@umit.maine.edu) and Jennifer A. Crittenden (E-mail: Jennifer.crittenden@ umit.main.edu) is a Research Associate, both at the University of Maine Center on Aging, 5723 D.P. Corbett Building, Orono, ME 04469.

[Haworth co-indexing entry note]: "Invention with Abused Older Males: Conceptual and Clinical Perspectives." Kaye, Lenard W., Diane Kay, and Jennifer A. Crittenden. Co-published simultaneously in *Journal of Elder Abuse & Neglect*™ (The Haworth Maltreatment & Trauma Press®, an imprint of The Haworth Press, Inc.) Vol. 19, No. 1/2, 2007, pp. 153-172; and: *Abuse of Older Men* (ed: Jordan I. Kosberg) The Haworth Maltreatment & Trauma Press®, an imprint of The Haworth Press, Inc., 2007, pp. 153-172. Single or multiple copies of this article are available for a fee from The Haworth Document Delivery Service [1-800-HAWORTH, 9:00 a.m. - 5:00 p.m. (EST). E-mail address: docdelivery@haworthpress.com].

INTRODUCTION

Older men experience mistreatment. As most elder abuse goes unreported, it is difficult to specify precise statistics that illustrate the magnitude of this problem. However, estimates indicate that between one and two million older Americans are victim to elder abuse, and older men make up one third of all victims of elder abuse (Westley, 2005). Though the incidence of abuse may be lower in older men than in older women, it is critical that practitioners working with older men understand the essential differences in the way that both genders experience and cope with abuse. They also need to understand the unique treatment needs of each gender. Such differences affect men's help seeking behavior, available treatments, treatment outcomes, and shape the overall treatment experience. Additionally, practitioners working with older men who experience mistreatment are faced with a wide range of issues including practical challenges, such as identifying abuse and selecting the most appropriate treatment modality, as well as relational issues affecting the interaction between client and service provider. The mental health issues that abused men face add further complexity to the clinical picture and serve to underscore the significance that gender can be expected to play in one's approach to clinical intervention.

KEY CONCEPTS

For the purposes of this discussion, older men are defined as those males who are 65 or more years of age. They may live alone or with family, a spouse, roommates, or a paid caregiver. They may reside in their own home, in an independent or assisted living program, in a hospital, or in an institutional setting. In many respects, there are as many types of living situations for older men as there are individual older men, given that each older man's experiences are uniquely his own.

Mistreatment

Mistreatment is defined by the National Research Council as "(a) intentional actions that cause harm or create a serious risk of harm (whether or not harm is intended) to a vulnerable elder by a caregiver or other person who stands in a trusting relationship to the elder or (b) failure by a caregiver to satisfy the elder's basic needs or protect the elder from harm" (as cited in Fulmer et al., 2005, p. 525). Westley (2005) incorporates seven dimensions of elder mistreatment when defining abuse: (1) Physical abuse; (2) Psychological or emotional abuse; (3) Financial or material abuse; (4) Neglect; (5) Self-neglect; (6) Sexual abuse; and (7) Other aspects. The preceding examples illustrate the disagreement that currently exists among scholars as to the preferred definition of elder mistreatment. Furthermore, definitions vary by context. Buri, Daly, Hartz, and Jogerst (2006) recognize this complexity, and the current debate, by questioning "whether abuse includes passive neglect as well as intentional neglect, whether self-neglect is considered a form of elder abuse, whether financial exploitation is included, and whether sexual abuse is treated as a subset of physical abuse or as a separate category" (p. 563). This complexity necessarily lends an ambiguous hue to the understanding of elder mistreatment. For the purposes of this discussion, mistreatment is defined as the experience of physical abuse, sexual abuse, emotional abuse, exploitation and/or neglect of those over the age of 65. Though self-neglect is considered by many to constitute a form of elder abuse, it will not be included in this discussion. Self-neglect continues to be controversial category within the elder abuse literature (Woolf, 1998). As it is often difficult to differentiate self-neglect from other mental health conditions, this article focuses on abuse and mistreatment at the hands of other people in a man's life.

Perpetrator Relationship to Victim

Simply stated, the perpetrator is the responsible party who brings harm to the elder experiencing mistreatment, whether that harm is intentional or unintentional. Yet the relationship also may introduce a host of complex and cross-cutting dynamics between victim and perpetrator. Research findings suggest that the perpetrator of elder abuse is more likely than not to be a relative of the older victim, or a paid or unpaid caregiver (Hybels et al., 2006; Kosberg & MacNeil, 2003). An understanding of the problem of elder abuse requires appreciation of the studies that have been carried out which consider the dynamics between victim and perpetrator. In good part, it may be the fragile balance between stress and risk within caregiving relationships that impacts vulnerability to abuse. This complex dynamic will be explored further as the discussion that follows unfolds.

Risk Factors

Numerous studies have been undertaken to determine risk of abuse to elders. Low socioeconomic status, social isolation, dementia, chronic health conditions, emergency room visits, childhood trauma and depression have all been shown to be positively associated with a greater risk of mistreatment (Schiamberg & Gans, 2000; Erlingsson, Carlson, & Saveman, 2003; Nahmiash, 2002; Buri, Daly, Hartz, 2006 & Jogerst, 2006).

Fulmer et al. (2005) separate risk factors into two constructs: risk and vulnerability. By examining the likelihood of abuse in this way, it is possible to separately consider those factors that come into play as either external (risk) or internal (vulnerability) facets of the relationship dynamic, helping to further understand the crucial locus of control as it relates to these factors. Suffice it to say, at this point, risk reduction efforts with older men should take into account the orientation (internal versus external) from which intervention work is best posed.

The recognition of risk factors which are associated with abuse have to some extent influenced a current call for providing the professional community with education and training to help combat elder mistreatment. This frequently includes teaching practitioners how to identify elders at risk of mistreatment through the utilization of both screening tools and awareness, and implementing these skills into practice (Cooper, Katona, Finne-Soveri, Topinkova, Carpenter, & Livingston, 2006; Westley, 2005).

The Controversy Simply Stated

Men have not historically been considered an oppressed group, and are thought to comprise the majority of perpetrators in abusive relationships. While often such scenarios are accurate, preconceived notions that relate to men as perpetrators or as the privileged sex may overshadow the mistreatment that many older men face and prevent them from seeking help or obtaining appropriate services when it is available.

THE CURRENT SERVICE SCENARIO

There currently exists little awareness of elder abuse as an issue, and particularly as a men's issue. Despite the reality of mistreatment of older men, there has yet to be an effort to publicly focus on its occurrence. Ricker Hamilton, who has worked for Adult Protective Services in the state of Maine since 1982, has informed the authors that about one third (33%) of all victims of elder mistreatment are estimated to be men, and has remained relatively constant for the past twenty years (R. Hamilton, personal communication, November 27, 2006). Research that serves to underscore the hidden nature of elder abuse estimates that only one in every fourteen cases of elder abuse are actually reported (Westley, 2005). Hamilton further notes, "Public service announcements on television inform us about child abuse, domestic violence, drugs, and cigarettes but exclude efforts to promote public awareness of elder abuse" (R. Hamilton, personal communication, November 27, 2006).

The populations that most frequently come to mind as victims of abuse are women and children, and these groups do face higher incidence of mistreatment. However, lack of awareness of abuse of elders, and of men in particular, severely limits the ability to provide these victims with needed, appropriate, and effective treatment. Emergency services for men as a victim group remain virtually nonexistent.

Gendered Service Traditions

One might argue that traditional social services are not configured with the needs of older men in mind. Research indicates that many more women than men are aware of what services are available, and are generally more likely to seek help (Barusch, 2000). Additionally, just as the number of older women far outweighs the number of older men, these women are the primary consumers of services, leading to the necessity of women-focused services and, thus, influencing the existence of female-centered therapeutic ideologies (Kaye & Crittenden, 2005). Unfortunately, this may become a vicious cycle if one considers the ramifications of this having negative impact on older men's willingness to reach out for help, ability to access such assistance, and subsequently receive interventions appropriate to their individual situations.

Ethical Considerations

Ethical matters also influence the course of service provision for older men who experience mistreatment. With such a large percentage of mistreatment experiences maintained in secrecy by the victim, what is to be done if a client discloses abuse but refuses help? If a client has developed a relationship of trust with a practitioner who betrays that trust by reporting the abuse, how is that likely to affect the practitioner/client relationship? Beaulieu and Leclerc (2006) identify a set of ethical dilemmas: confidentiality versus collaboration, assessing responsibility, and the balance of competing values. These ethical issues further complicate the task of providing treatment to older men who experience mistreatment.

Certainly, stories of elder mistreatment provoke strong feelings within oneself as a person and as a practitioner. While few victims reach out for assistance after experiencing abuse, those who do may inadvertently pose ethical dilemmas for the practitioners who work with them. The responsibility to report under mandated reporting laws can at times create conflict with a client's autonomy and right to self-determination (Linzer, 2004). Do you withhold the report at clients' request because doing so will allow them to further control their own circumstance? Or do you report in hopes that such action will serve the clients' best interest? There are certainly cases where the decision to report will be quite clear. However, what is less clear are those circumstances that exist within the "gray area" of such laws. In all circumstances, practitioners are encouraged to discuss potential elder abuse with supervisors, trusted colleagues, or contacts within Adult Protective Services. While seeking out such input will not relinquish your duties under mandatory reporting laws, it will serve to provide you with a sounding board and allow you to see the situation outside of the context of your own personal feelings and biases. In addition, as Linzer notes, there are times when a keen therapeutic decision can be made in such cases that does not compromise the client's self determination nor the practitioner's responsibility to protect their client.

Lessons from the Veterans' Administration (VA)

There are some key principles of practice that can be gleaned from professionals within the VA who provide services to older men. As a service system, the VA is often called upon to provide services and treatment to a diverse group of men who all share the common experience of military service (some during wartime). These life events may, in some ways, increase group cohesiveness, facilitate the nature of the group and individual treatments provided to them.

Darrin Sanford-Rocket, LCSW, of the Maine Veteran's Administration, explains that older men who access mental health services through the VA are likely to do so as a result of recommendations from other veterans who have previously accessed services. In her experience, there appears to be great acceptance by older men of seeking help through the VA, and she suggests that some of the stigma of accessing help may be lessened by the knowledge that, as veterans, they gave to their country, and the VA services are something that they have earned and are less likely to be viewed as a "handout." VA facilities recognize the importance of each veteran's contribution to their country, making veterans more likely to access services through VA settings than non-veterans through non-VA community based services. Nonetheless, few reports of elder mistreatment are made to VA social workers (D. Sanford-Rocket, personal communication, November 27, 2006). It is not clear if this is because veterans experience less abuse than other older men, or if veterans as a group, similar to their non-veteran counterparts, find it difficult to disclose their mistreatment.

Lessons from Adult Protective Services (APS)

Community APS workers, on a daily basis, are called upon to address elder mistreatment, yet face a dearth of resources to offer their clients. Ricker Hamilton describes the job of APS personnel as "working in isolation" without an established network of service providers and indicates that workers are "left alone to make magic." On a federal level, there is no mandate regarding elder abuse, which reflects the low priority assigned elder abuse as a political "hot topic," and the lack of public awareness (R. Hamilton, personal communication, November 27, 2006). While elder abuse is generally underreported, it may also be assumed that this is even more so true for older men. For those older men in need of shelter, it is often difficult to find them emergency shelter. For older men at risk of abuse in their homes, there is commonly nowhere for these men to go. APS workers are thus left with no options to place an older man experiencing mistreatment. With this in mind, a clinician may face unique challenges in finding a safe environment for the older man who has been mistreated. Medical issues may further reduce the number of viable housing options for one's client. Likewise, clinicians face a system that is not accustomed to working with older men who have been the victims of mistreatment (R. Hamilton, personal communication, November 27, 2006).

OLDER MEN AND HELP SEEKING

Socialization of Men

Though it is difficult to discuss the traits of men without feeding into gender stereotypes, there are certain aspects of masculinity which, when applied to the experience of men (particularly older men), can be expected to affect their help seeking behaviors. The culture of masculinity in the US is one that underscores the qualities of strength and self-sufficiency. Men are expected to be breadwinners, and take care of others through providing financially and materially. Men are given messages like "boys don't cry" in their formative years, and are encouraged to suppress their emotions and discouraged from talking about their feelings, as it could be interpreted as a sign of weakness. Of course, men can deeply feel emotion, but the societal expectation of being strong and unwavering impacts their ability to freely express such feelings.

These traits of masculinity are embedded in older males of the pre-baby boom generation. There is a stigma attached to seeking help, it flies in the face of such "stiff upper lip" mentality messages to "tough it out" or "raise yourself up by your bootstraps" that so many older men had been raised to embrace. As the baby boomers begin to age and enter older adulthood, there may be a shift in the help seeking behaviors of men, as there is expected to be less of a help-seeking stigma among this cohort (Barusch, 2000).

Older Men and Help Seeking

Societal (and self-imposed) expectations of male-centered behavior continue to have a negative effect on the ability of older men to seek help. Services may be confidential, but acknowledging emotional problems and seeking help for them may make a man doubt his masculinity, and be viewed as an admission of weakness or dependency. This ingrained stigma, that precludes inclinations to seek assistance, creates a powerful barrier for men accessing services (Barusch, 2000). Additionally, as mental health problems may manifest physical symptoms (i.e., sleeplessness, shortness of breath, headaches), older men may decide not to seek help for these symptoms for fear of being diagnosed with a physical condition that could limit their independence. The threat of losing independence and being placed in care is a very real fear for many older men. So, in addition to the stigma associated with seeking help, many professionals also must work against the perception that once an older adult discloses abuse, they will be forced out of their homes and lose control over their lives. For older adults who live independently, the thought of leaving one's home can be devastating. The idea of losing one's independence may, in the client's eyes, be worse than living with ongoing mistreatment (Beaulieu & Leclerc, 2006).

When trauma is experienced, coping mechanisms that a man experiences may further keep him from seeking formal help. Daughtry and Paulk (2006) suggest that while men and women do share some similarities between them with regard to coping behaviors, there are also some notable differences. Their research found that women are more likely to seek professional help as a coping mechanism whereas men, unlike women, are more likely to identify instrumental distraction (sports, computer activities, reading, etc.) as a coping mechanism. Male participants in the Daughtry and Paulk (2006) study also identified drinking to intoxication and experimenting with drugs as two negative coping strategies that are unique to men.

Thus, clinicians need to be sensitive to the coping strategies that their clients develop with regard to trauma. Fostering positive coping strategies for men may include a number of outlets, even some that may not typically come to mind, such as seeking support from family and friends; self-enhancing strategies such as increasing self-esteem, trying a new routine, or healthy eating; and cognitive strategies such as recalling positive memories, engaging in long-term planning, and focusing on immediate options in one's life (Daughtry & Paulk, 2006).

Negative coping strategies must be addressed as soon as possible with male clients as older men are at higher risk than older women for substance abuse and suicide. The combination of trauma and loss can likewise become a breeding ground for adverse coping strategies. After the loss of a spouse, older men are much more likely to die during the first year of bereavement than women (Barusch, 2000). In men's marital relationships, spouses generally provide older men with their primary sources of emotional support and social connections. When an older man's spouse dies, the male is left with a void in these areas, and men that are not able to seek help to gain outside support may suffer.

Essentials of Practice with Older Men

How do practitioners use what they know to reach out to older men and make them more receptive to receiving help? How can men be encouraged to get beyond the stigma of seeking help so that they may help themselves? Barusch (2000) suggests finding ways of encouraging older men to participate in services that are congruent with their personal goals. Older men may feel better about their help seeking if they are invested in the outcome and are able to identify personal goals that are seen to be realistic and attainable.

Older men often find groups to be a more approachable way of seeking treatment (Barusch, 2000). The dynamics of group work remove the responsibility of the helping relationship from the practitioner, and give it to the group members. In fact, it has been found that older men gain a great deal of satisfaction through helping their group members (Kaye & Applegate, 1993). Additionally, the opportunity to help others (rather than helping oneself) is often seen as a motivator for men to join groups (Barusch, 2000). Helping others with their problems can give older men insight in the ways to solve their own problems which, in turn, improves self-esteem.

Multi-systemic therapeutic interventions have been utilized more frequently in practice, particularly with youth and families. Applegate (2000) discusses the benefit of multi-systemic work with older men. The multi-systemic model examines the role of the individual as he interacts with all others in the system. Systems include micro (one-on-one relationships), mezzo (small groups and families), and macro (large organizations and society) entities. Working on improving an older man's experience in each system, self-identified short term goals are achieved. This creates an opportunity to build on successes and makes men more open to subsequent short-term, goal-oriented interventions.

Keeping in mind the particular needs of older men with regard to treatment (as well as individual needs), practitioners work toward providing treatment interventions that reflect the "best fit" for the needs of their older male clients. Treatment is best approached through a combination of solid theory, practice knowledge, and respect for the client. However, here too, there are differences in the way men and women perceive concepts such as respect within the clinical relationship. Findings from the Scheyett and McCarthy study (2006) of men and women with mental illness suggest that women most often define respect as a provider's willingness to enter into an "understanding" and "caring" therapeutic relationship and place a high value on the importance of being understood by their clinician. On the other hand, for men with mental illness, respect is often defined by a therapist who listens to his client and who also engages in mutual information exchange. Independence within the therapeutic relationship is also a key component of respect as defined by male clients (Scheyett & McCarthy).

TYPES OF TREATMENT AND OUTCOMES WITH OLDER MEN

If you are a clinician, vigilance will likely be your best therapeutic tool. The older men you treat may not come to you with a presenting issue of mistreatment, and even once a trusting therapeutic relationship is formed, an older male client still may not disclose mistreatment. Rather, you may be seeing a client for a variety of reasons including bereavement, substance abuse, posttraumatic stress disorder, depression, and health-related issues, among others. Mistreatment is often an underlying problem or an unacknowledged experience. Thus your treatment may have a dual focus: managing the symptoms of the presenting issue while also screening for, identifying, and subsequently addressing the mistreatment or abuse that has been experienced.

Treatment Settings Utilized by Older Men

Group settings. These settings have been shown to be a highly effective treatment modality for older adults, especially men. Such modalities capitalize on the therapeutic power of individuals with commonalities joining together to share their experiences. The group dynamic allows for open sharing in a safe environment, and group members lend support to each other to help solve problems (Yalom, 1995). Haringsma, Engels, Van Der Leeden, and Spinhoven (2006) studied the effectiveness of using the "coping with depression" (CWD) educational course as a strategy for teaching coping methods for depression in older persons. They found that the course evidenced measurable benefit to participants' levels of depression and participants were able to sustain this level of improvement for an average period of 14 months following the completion of the course. Another effective group work model shown to be effective with older men is the self-help group, particularly 12-step programs such as Alcoholics Anonymous (AA).

It has been observed (Barusch, 2000) that men are more likely to join a group with an educational theme as opposed to a therapeutic one. The outcome of treatment may be the same; however, the manner in which treatment is presented can make a difference in the ability of a client to incorporate change in his life. In an educational group, a client may feel more in control; also it situates the group within the context of learning skill acquisition and accumulation of information as opposed to "fixing" pathology.

Literature suggests that mixed gender therapy groups may not be as effective as more homogeneous men's groups (Ogrodniczuk, 2006). If a mixed gendered group is utilized, a clinician may be best advised to have a sufficient number of men in the group to allow individual males to have the opportunity to gain a sense of comradery with others of perceived "like mind," thus providing a pathway toward gender-sensitive contextual privacy. In such cases, men are enabled to form a smaller "sub group," should that be sought (Ogrodniczuk).

Individual therapy. Research on individual therapy with older men has shown that they are less likely to enter into a psychotherapeutic relationship. However, for those who display a willingness to enter into such treatment, there appear to be particular forms of therapy that one should consider: Life review and narrative therapy approaches.

Draucker (2003) found that narrative therapy and related techniques may serve to enhance treatment outcomes for men. Specifically, many men are able to reformulate trauma stories (including abuse) within their lives into more positive narratives. Many times, survivors of trauma will have difficulty experiencing and labeling their own emotions. For men, this is particularly possible. Draucker found that men who had survived trauma often tell the story of a time when they were successfully able to feel sadness, joy, or compassion for the first time since experiencing trauma. When male clients are able to successfully reformulate their narrative they may begin, for the first time, to talk about or view their outcome. Consequently, they are able to recognize "normal" emotions or they are successful in identifying a pivotal moment where they were able to "awake" from the feelings that they had been facing as a result of their trauma. Draucker suggests that such resurgence stories, as they emerge in therapy, reflect a personal "reaction against the societal expectation that men should discount their feelings" (Draucker, p. 13).

Draucker (2003) presents several narrative tools that can be used with male trauma survivors including point of view questions, different context questions, and different time frame questions. Point of view questions ask the client how others may have viewed his actions, allowing him to safely step out of his own point of view and begin to rewrite his narrative. Different context questions ask the client to discuss contexts that are not a part of the problem narrative. Such questions entail identifying the places where he feels safe, or at peace, or simply contexts that do not play a part of the trauma experience. Different time frame questions allow the client to identify times in his life, or even during a typical day, when trauma is not present or is not dominating his actions or thoughts. Such times might include when he is with his grandchildren or when he is at work. All of these questions help to build a new narrative about one's life and explore times and contexts that are not colored by the mistreatment he has experienced. Working against cultural and social expectations of what a "man" is willing to confront adds challenges to this work with abused men.

Ogrodniczuk's (2006) review of clinical outcomes for men versus women in short term individual therapy confirms that women do better in supportive type therapies that are characterized by empathy, affiliation, and affective expression. Male clients tend to realize better outcomes in interpretive therapies that are categorized by a therapeutic relationship allowing for emotional distance and independence. This is particularly true of treatment for depressive symptoms.

Another individual therapeutic treatment model that could be useful in working with older men is de Shazer's (1988) solution-focused therapy. This model utilizes tools such as "exceptions," "reframing," and the "miracle question" to encourage clients in treatment to view whatever negative situations they may be experiencing in a different, more positive light. This model is empowering for clients in treatment, as the therapist guides the client to find his personal solutions, unique to his own experience. The ways that solution-focused therapy may be utilized in treating older men will be discussed further in the discussion of diagnoses and treatment.

Community-based treatment. The community-based modality of treatment is earning validation as an effective tool for use with various client populations. Richman, Wilson, Scally, Edwards and Wood (2003) present evidence of the effectiveness of providing outreach treatment to older adults. They profile the impact of an outreach support team that provides interim mental health treatment to clients who are waiting for inpatient psychiatric care. Six out of nine men who received this service remained at home and did not require psychiatric admission once a bed became available (Richman et al.). Community-based treatment also has been identified by APS workers to be a needed resource for isolated older male clients (R. Hamilton, personal communication, November 27, 2006). Outreach services may have a number of advantages over services based in a clinical setting. When service providers come to an older person's home, the stigma associated with appearing in public and seeking help is avoided. Also, for older men with mobility limitations, home-based care removes the necessity of obtaining transportation to services. Finally, an older man meeting with a clinician in his home is on "his own turf," in a more comfortable, familiar environment, and not in an office that may potentially be unfamiliar, sterile, and–ultimately–quite threatening.

Diagnoses treated. Older men may seek treatment for a number of different reasons. Some of the most frequent include substance abuse, bereavement, and depression. When an older man seeks treatment for a mental health issue, a lifetime of factors need to be considered in order to provide the most effective treatment, including prior trauma, current problems, and co-occurring conditions/dual diagnosis.

TYPES OF CLINICAL TREATMENTS
AND THEIR OUTCOMES

Post Traumatic Stress Disorder (PTSD)

PTSD is the most often observed diagnosis in veterans and other survivors of war. As the baby boomers age, Vietnam veterans can be expected to represent larger proportions of the older men accessing Veteran's Administration services. The occurrence of PTSD in older individuals may either be delayed onset, chronic and either previously or recently diagnosed, or reemerge after having been in remission. Aarts and Op Den Velde (1996) present a case in which a Dutch Veteran from WWII experienced trauma while captured during wartime and was diagnosed with PTSD upon his return, and experienced flashbacks for five years. He was then symptom-free for several years until experiencing another episode of flashbacks, lasting another three years, that had been triggered by news reports of war in which his son was a soldier. His third episode of PTSD occurred after being in an auto accident when his symptoms of PTSD appeared again, but diminished after participating in a Veteran's group. This experience is an example of the "sinewy nature" of PTSD. A diagnosis of PTSD in remission may be triggered and then return to the surface after experiencing another trauma later in life. It is the clinician's role, when working with older men, to be aware of the client's past trauma history. Though the client may be asymptomatic, it is important to know this in the event of a future trauma. Indeed, the experience of powerlessness felt by a mistreated older man could lead to subsequent trauma that "triggers" PTSD symptoms.

Depression and Bereavement

Another diagnosis frequently treated in older men is depression, resulting often from bereavement (commonly associated with the loss of a spouse) or from other factors associated with old age. Norton et al. (2006) found that both older men and women experience thoughts of suicide; older men face higher risk of actually committing suicide.

Solution-focused treatment, originally created by de Shazer (1988), may be particularly useful to clinicians in working with older men who experience depression. Feelings of hopelessness, low self-worth, and lack of empowerment experienced by older men with depression can be reframed to be seen in a more positive light. The tool of "exceptions" asks a client to recall a positive exception to their negative experience.

For example, if an older man talks about how he is frustrated by his lack of mobility and declining independence, how he cannot do anything for himself anymore, it would be the role of the therapist to encourage the client to identify those moments (exceptions) when he does feel independent and is able to do things for himself. So, too, the client will be asked to consider ways that those experiences and feelings can be replicated. In using the "miracle question," the therapist posits this general probe: "Suppose you go to bed at night and, while you are sleeping and unbeknownst to you, a miracle occurs overnight. When you awake in the morning, your life is better. How will you know? What has changed?" This method can be a way to encourage "outside the box" problem solving with clients, and a technique for instilling hope for change. The "miracle" allows clients to view their future life in a positive manner, and it is their vision of a changed future that is instrumental in moving forward. It is this "co-manufacturing" of hope that is established in the helping relationship which is essential to the creation of positive change.

Additionally, encouraging older men to develop a support network, either through social activities, strengthening family relationships, or by means of therapeutic/educational groups is essential in treating older men for depression. These positive relationships reduce isolation, which in turn impacts resiliency.

Substance Abuse

It is well documented that the experience of trauma and substance abuse are often closely associated. As such, it is recommended that clinicians treat the underlying experience of trauma along with the possibility of substance abuse. Williams et al. (2005) promote both respectful and empathetic counseling that offers older adults options to minimize their intake of abused substances. This approach often involves group therapies that focus on the issues that bring on alcohol abuse. For example, Sedlack, Doheny, Estok, and Zeller (2000) found that women often benefited more from group support to increase self-esteem and address issues of vulnerability, while men need to focus on issues of weakness, dependency, and self-sacrifice. According to Barrick and Connors (2002), older persons will often experience relapse because of intrapersonal issues, such as a negative emotional state, than interpersonal issues such as pressure from peers. Professionals should focus on helping older adults cope with intrapersonal issues without the use of alcohol. Intrapersonal issues include "a supportive, non-confrontational approach, building skills to cope with negative emotions (e.g., loss, loneliness), rebuilding a social support network, and offering appropriate medical and social service linkages" (Barrick & Connors, 2002, p. 588).

Other Issues

In addition to the systemic challenges that impact the constellation of services available to older men, and their accessibility, service providers have other factors to take into account which affect their interactions with older male clients and their ability to form beneficial helping relationships. Such factors may influence the ability for practitioners to work successfully with older male clients. Personal attributes of therapists such as age and sex/gender can impact this relationship, and maintaining an awareness of possible counter transference issues is essential to the development of successful helping relationships.

RECOMMENDATIONS

Redesigning the Intervention System

In order for the needs of older men who experience mistreatment to be more effectively integrated within existing social service systems, a number of changes are needed. First and foremost, public awareness surrounding elder abuse must become a priority. Until there is adequate awareness to change the depth and breadth of current service provisions, the needs of older men will continue to go unmet. Agencies and individual service providers need to learn how to more effectively identify older men who may be at risk of mistreatment. Students preparing for careers in the helping professions need to acquire the skills required for elder abuse screening. Such expertise will best be acquired if it is formally integrated into educational programs of the social work, nursing, medical, and associated mental health professions. Practitioners on the front lines of clinical practice require "retooling." Building a relationship of trust with clients will encourage regular discussion with older clients during appointments about the care that they receive and their relationships with caregivers. Training of informal supports is an option worthy of consideration and may be carried out in the community with those who come into contact with older men on a regular basis, such as barbers, clergy and church members, public utility workers, volunteers, and postal carriers. Fundamental changes in the way services are provided to older men will allow practitioners to identify individuals at risk, and permit them to address situations at a preventative level.

Staffing and Training

As the number of older Americans continues to grow, practitioners will work with an increasing number of older men. By increasing the skill set that is applicable to the needs of older men, practitioners will be able to prepare themselves to be able to work more effectively with their older male clients. Integrating awareness of risk to elders for possible mistreatment, and considering these risks throughout treatment will aid in implementing effective preventative measures and safety plans. Additionally, service providers should be constantly striving to attain more information regarding effective treatment models to use in practice with clients.

Implications for Practice

Group work, fostering trust in working relationships with clients, showing respect for each man's experience, utilization of multidisciplinary teams and customized, gender-sensitive outreach methods should be utilized in future practice with older men. Paying close attention to each man's particular therapeutic needs and responses to treatment is also important.

More research is needed in the realm of gendered services and treatment models. There exists a dearth of literature focusing on not only mistreatment of older men but also the treatment modalities that are most effective in addressing this issue. Older men continue to challenge service systems in ways that the field is not yet prepared to address. Investigating the use of innovative techniques for reaching men, including the use of medical providers and other gatekeepers, is needed. Further research into applying community-based services models to treatment of older persons and the use of multidisciplinary teams continue to represent an exciting prospect to consider for future interventions with abused older men.

A Look Toward the Future

With the importance of cultural competence being a core value in many applied professions, there is a need to consider viewing practice with older men through the lens of a "culture of masculinity." This is necessary in order to provide older men with services that are sensitive to their needs. A practitioner that provides services to older clients with consideration of this culture and its impact on older men will be much better equipped to provide meaningful, appropriate, and effective treatment to the older men that they serve.

REFERENCES

Aarts, P.G.H., & Op den Velde, W. (1996). Prior traumatization and the process of aging: Theory and clinical implications. In B.A van der Kolk, A.C. McFarlane, & L. Weisaeth, (Eds.), *Traumatic stress: The effects of overwhelming experience on mind, body, and society* (pp. 359-377). New York: Guilford Press.

Abeles, N., Cooley, S., Deitch, I.M., Harper, M.S., Hinrichsen, G., Lopez, M.A., & Molinari, V.A. (1998). *What practitioners should know about working with older adults*. American Psychological Association. Washington, DC.

Applegate, J.W. (2000). Conceptualizing the experience of older men: Implications for practice. *Geriatric Care Management Journal, 10*(1), 6-10.

Barrick, C., & Connors, G. J. (2002). Relapse prevention and maintaining abstinence in older adults with alcohol abuse disorders. *Drugs and Aging, 19*(8), 583-594.

Barusch, A.S. (2000). Serving older men: Dilemmas and opportunities for geriatric care managers. *Geriatric Care Management Journal, 10*(1), 31-37.

Beaulieu, M., & Leclerc, N. (2006). Ethical and psychosocial issues raised by the practice in cases of mistreatment of older adults. *Journal Gerontological Social Work, 46*(3/4), 161-186.

Buri, H., Daly, J.M., Hartz, A.J., & Jogerst, G.J. (2006). Factors associated with self-reported elder mistreatment in Iowa's frailest elders. *Research on Aging, 28*(5), 562-581.

Cooper, C.C., Katona, C., Finne-Soveri, H., Topinkova, E., Carpenter, G.I., & Livingston, G. (2006). Indicators of elder abuse: A cross-national comparison of psychiatric morbidity and other determinants in the ad-hoc study. *American Journal of Geriatric Psychiatry, 14*(6), 489-497.

Daughtry, D., & Paulk, D.L. (2006). Gender differences in depression-related coping patterns. *Counseling and Clinical Psychology Journal, 3*(2), 46-59.

de Shazer, S. (1985). *Keys to solution in brief therapy*. New York: Norton.

Draucker, C.B. (2003). Unique outcomes of women and men who were abused. *Perspectives in Psychiatric Care, 39*(1), 7-16.

Erlingsson, C.L., Carlson, S.L., & Saveman, B. (2003). Elder abuse risk indicators and screening questions: Results from a literature search and a panel of experts from developed and developing countries. In E. Podnieks, J.I. Kosberg, & A. Lowenstein (Eds.), *Elder abuse: Selected papers from the Prague World Conference on Family Violence.* (pp. 185-203). Binghamton, NY: Haworth Press.

Fulmer, T., Paveza, G., VandeWeerd, C., Fairchild, S., Guadagno, L., Bolton-Blatt, M., & Norman, R. (2005). Dyadic vulnerability and risk profiling for elder neglect. *The Gerontologist, 45*(4), 525-534.

Haringsma, R., Engels, G.I., Van Der Leeden, R., & Spinhoven, P. (2006). Predictors of response to the "Coping with Depression" course for older adults. A field study. *Aging and Mental Health, 10*(4), 424-434.

Hybels, C.F., Blazer, D.G., Pieper, C.F., Burchett, B.M., Hays, J.C., Fillenbaum, G.G., Kubzansky, L.D., & Berkman, L.F. (2006). Sociodemographic characteristics of the neighborhood and depressive symptoms in older adults: Using multilevel modeling in geriatric psychiatry. *American Journal of Geriatric Psychiatry, 14*(6), 498-506.

Kaye, L.W., & Applegate, J.S. (1993). Family support groups for male caregivers: Benefits of participation. *Journal of Gerontological Social Work, 20*(3/4), 167-185.

Kaye, L.W., & Crittenden, J.A.(2005). Principles of clinical practice with older men. *Journal of Sociology and Social Welfare, 32*(1), 99-123.

Kosberg, J.I., & MacNeil, G. (2003). The elder abuse of custodial grandparents: A hidden phenomenon. In E. Podnieks, J.I., Kosberg, & A. Lowenstein (Eds.), *Elder abuse: Selected papers from the Prague World Conference on Family Violence* (pp.33-53). Binghamton, NY: Haworth Press.

Linzer, N. (2004). An ethical dilemma in elder abuse. *Journal of Gerontological Social Work, 43* (2/3), 165-173.

Nahmiash, D. (2002). Powerlessness and abuse and neglect of older adults. *Journal of Elder Abuse & Neglect, 14*(1), 21-47.

Norton, M.C., Skoog, I., Toone, L., Corcoran, C., Tschanz, J.T., Lisota, R.D., Hart, A.D., Zandi, P.P., Breitner, J.C.S., Welsh-Bohmer, K.A., & Steffans, D.C. (2006). Three year incidence of first-onset depressive syndrome in a population sample of older adults: The Cache county study. *American Journal of Geriatric Psychiatry, 14*(3), 237-245.

Ogrodniczuk, J.S. (2006). Men, women and their outcome in psychotherapy, *Psychotherapy Research, 16*(4), 453-462.

Richman, A., Wilson, K., Scally, L., Edwards, P., & Wood, J. (2003). Service innovations: An outreach support team for older people with mental illness–crisis intervention. *Psychiatric Bulletin, 27,* 348-351.

Scheyett, A.M., & McCarthy, E. (2006). Women and men with mental illnesses: Voicing different service needs. *Afflia: Journal of Women and Social Work, 21*(4), 407-418.

Schiamberg, L.B., & Gans, D. (2000). Elder abuse by adult children: An applied ecological framework for understanding contextual risk factors and the intergenerational character of quality of life. *International Journal of Aging and Human Development, 50*(4), 329-359.

Sedlack, C.A., Doheny, M., Estok, P.J., & Zeller, R.A. (2000). Alcohol use in women 65 years of age and older. *Health Care of Women International, 21,* 567-581.

Simpson, C., & De Silva, P. (2003). Service interventions: Multi-disciplinary team assessments: A method of improving the quality and accessibility of old age psychiatry services. *Psychiatric Bulletin, 27,* 346-348.

van Etten, D. (2006). Psychotherapy with older adults: Benefits and barriers. *Journal of Psychological Nursing and Mental Health Services, 44*(11), 28-33.

Weeks, L.E., Richards, J.L., Nilsson, T., Kozma, A., & Bryanton, O. (2004). A gendered analysis of the abuse of older adults: Evidence from professionals. *Journal of Elder Abuse & Neglect, 16*(2), 1-15.

Westley, C. (2005). Elder mistreatment: Self-learning module. *MEDSURG Nursing,* *14*(2), 133-137.

Wilcox, B.J. (2006). *Men who avoid certain risk factors in midlife may have longer, healthier life.* American Medical Association (AMA). Retrieved November 17, 2006 from http://www.newswise.com/p/articles/view/525137/

Williams, J.M., Ballard, M.B. & Alessi, H. (2005). Aging and alcohol abuse: Increasing counselor awareness. *ADULTSPAN Journal, 4*(1), 7-18.

Woolf, L.M. (1998). *Elder abuse and neglect.* Retrieved December 11, 2006 from http://www.webster.edu/~woolflm/abuse.html#neglect

Yaffe, K., & Steffans, D. (2006). Epidemiology of mental health: A keystone of geriatric psychiatry. *American Journal of Geriatric Psychiatry, 14*(6), 477-479.

Yalom, I.D. (1995). *The theory and practice of group psychotherapy* (4th ed.). New York: Basic Books.

doi:10.1300/J084v19n01_10

Abuse of Elderly Male Clients: Efforts and Experiences in Rural and Urban Adult Protective Services

Robert Blundo, PhD, LCSW

Joseph Bullington, CSM

SUMMARY. Elder abuse has not been viewed as seriously as child abuse because of the emotional sensibilities attached to child abuse. Although elder abuse is experienced disproportionately by women, men also are in need of protection and engagement. An important factor for understanding the work with elderly men is the social construction of manhood. Both urban and rural settings recognize this as a significant starting point to engage men in services. This paper describes the efforts in both rural and urban Adult Protective Service agencies to identify and work with abused elderly men from a strengths and solution-focused perspective. doi:10.1300/J084v19n01_11 *[Article copies available for a fee from The Haworth Document Delivery Service: 1-800-HAWORTH. E-mail address: <docdelivery@haworthpress.com> Website: <http://www.HaworthPress.com> © 2007 by The Haworth Press, Inc. All rights reserved.]*

Robert Blundo is Professor, Department of Social Work at the University of North Carolina Wilmington, Wilmington, NC 28403 (E-mail: blunder@uncw.edu). Joseph Bullington is the Director of the Department of Health and Human Resources, Wyoming County District, Pineville, WV 24874 (E-mail: jbullington@wvdhhr.org).

[Haworth co-indexing entry note]: "Abuse of Elderly Male Client: Efforts and Experiences in Rural and Urban Adult Protective Services." Blundo, Robert, and Joseph Bullington. Co-published simultaneously in *Journal of Elder Abuse & Neglect™* (The Haworth Maltreatment & Trauma Press®, an imprint of The Haworth Press, Inc.) Vol. 19, No. 1/2, 2007, pp. 173-191; and: *Abuse of Older Men* (ed: Jordan I. Kosberg) The Haworth Maltreatment & Trauma Press®, an imprint of The Haworth Press, Inc., 2007, pp. 173-191. Single or multiple copies of this article are available for a fee from The Haworth Document Delivery Service [1-800-HAWORTH, 9:00 a.m. - 5:00 p.m. (EST). E-mail address: docdelivery@haworthpress.com].

doi:10.1300/J084v19n01_11

KEYWORDS. Elder abuse, men, solution-focused, rural, urban, masculinity

But yet, before thou prosecute the act,
Show him the letter which my sister sent;
There let him read his own indictment first,
And then proceed to execution.

King Lear, William Shakespeare

Ragan plots the murder of her father, King Lear, at the hands of the messenger in Shakespeare's play from 1605 and thus has it been down through the ages. Family members and caregivers have taken advantage and have abused other family members including vulnerable elderly relatives. Although a part of the human condition, it has not been until recently that elder abuse has been taken seriously as a social problem. Even though elder abuse does not command the same emotional sensibilities as child abuse in American society, it has become a focus of intervention for human service agencies. Both ageism and genderism have played a part in the slowness with which elder abuse services have developed.

INTRODUCTION

For women and men alike, ageism has left the elderly disregarded and discredited as a group (Aitken & Griffin, 1996). In a time dominated by youthfulness, ageing is something to be avoided in many ways. In her research on elder abuse, Pritchard (2001) found that workers themselves are prone to express this avoidance by not providing the in-depth services for the elderly as they might children. The report, *Ageism in America*, written for the 2005 White House Conference on Aging (International Longevity Center, 2005), describes ageism in every facet of American life for people over 65. The 2006 federal budget for elder abuse prevention and adult protective services placed a funding freeze on major existing programs. Yet, the report described the depth of discrimination in the areas of healthcare, nursing homes, emergency services, and workplace as represented in the media, advertisement and marketing (International Longevity Center).

Gender differences are considerable in terms of reported and non-reported elder abuse. The 1996 National Victim Assistance Academy report noted that variations in terms of definitions of what constitutes elder abuse and the nature of the reporting make it difficult to provide exacting figures (National Victim Assistance Academy, 1996). For example, some studies not only use different age groups for elderly but might not include self-neglect. In the statistical overview, the Academy estimated that approximately 1.8 million elders are victims of various forms of abuse, including self-neglect, each year. In terms of substantiation, the Academy reported that 54.9% of all reports were substantiated and 54.9% of those cases were self-neglect cases. Elderly males made up approximately 37.9% of these substantiated cases and of these approximately 37.6% were substantiated as self-neglect cases. Importantly, many women and men never reported incidences of abuse and men were 11% less likely to report being abused. The National Elder Abuse Incidence Study (National Center on Elder Abuse, 1998) reported that in 1996 of persons age 60 and over, men were the majority (62.2%) of victims of abandonment in substantiated cases which was, in general, the reverse of other categories where women made up roughly two-thirds of the substantiated cases. This finding as well as other abuses might relate to Kosberg's (1998) notion that neglect and abuse may represent a "pay back" by members of the family who had been abused by the elder man when he was younger. This study also found that 89.7% of perpetrators in substantiated cases were family members, of which 47.3% were adult children and 19.3% were spouses. It is interesting to note that in these two major reports, the statistics for men had to be inferred from incident reports for elderly females under specific abuse categories.

The focus of this article does not in any way intend to challenge the fact that women, in general, and elderly women, in particular, are most often victims of abuse; this is not being disputed in any way. The abuse of women has been and continues to be a most serious problem facing our society and a serious challenge facing those services attempting to address the problems of women. Yet, we need to make an effort to recognize that elderly men are potential victims as well. Those males who come to the attention of service providers need as much attention and care as do female victims.

It is the intention of this inquiry to describe the types of male elder abuse reported in both urban and rural settings and the approaches to services taken by workers in both settings. Adult Protective Service (APS) workers in social service agencies in rural Appalachia, as well as such workers in urban settings, were interviewed over a period of four months. APS workers were asked to consider their experiences with men 60 or older in terms of the types of reports, who made the reports, the experiences they have had or are having with elderly men in the course of their investigations, findings and day-to-day work with these men. The results of their documentation and interviews have been compiled and evaluated by the authors to better understand the way in which male elder abuse is being reported, the types of abuse reported, and the methods used by APS workers in engaging and assisting abused elderly men. The discussion begins with the very notion of what it means to be a "man" in our culture and its impact on our study findings.

"BEING A MAN":
IMPLICATIONS FOR ELDERLY MALE ABUSE

I had a report about a man once because no one had seen him for a while. When I made it up the camp road, I found his house with weeds over my head and it was hard to make it to the door. I have a tough stomach, but when I finally convinced him I needed to talk with him and got him to open the door, I had to step back and ask him to come outside. He had not shaved or bathed for a very long time and he had seven dogs living in the house with him. He would just dump the food in the middle of the room and they would go to it. There was little that I could do at that time since he was articulate and competent. (story from Appalachia)

It is important to briefly reflect on the notion of "manhood" and its consequence for men, their caretakers and the social service workers. The social construction of the notion of what it is to "be a man" generally has as part of the belief system that men do not cry or complain and are able to take care of themselves in tough situations. In addition, we find the general trend that men do not complain or share issues with others. Real men are seen to be stoic providers who do not need help from others. The consequences are increased health hazards, as they wait until symptoms have persisted to a point of severe health crisis. Evidence shows that the gap in longevity is more than biology between men and women. Sabo's (2004) review of the literature points to "social and cultural factors related to lifestyle, gender identity, and behavior" (p. 321) as important factors as well as race, sexual orientation and socioeconomic factors. Society in both its dominant and marginalized constructs of masculinities support this construction of what men internalize and maintain as a supra identity of manhood.

The societal portrayal of men reflects the idea of proper "manliness" as being strong, independent and competent. Cook (1997) notes that the news media's bias in reporting cases of men being abused corresponds to our society's notion that men who are abused or mistreated are "wimps" to be ridiculed. He gives the example of a headline for an article describing a woman's attempt to kill her husband for his insurance. The lead story title read: "Husband Survives the Lumps and Bumps of a New Marriage" (Cook, p. 127). Likewise, the consequence of the Lorena Bobbitt case, where she cut off the penis of her husband in 1993, led to a flood of jokes on prime time television and in offices and even within social agencies. If this had been the story of a man who had mutilated his wife, the story would have gotten less press and would not have been seen as humorous.

The elderly men involved in this research effort were born prior to 1946 and grew up in a different gendered world than now exists. They came to adulthood in the early to late 1940s through the 1960s. Many have worked from an early age and few in either the urban or rural settings had completed higher education. These men have defined themselves through socialization into American and regional constructions of manhood that they have lived out over the past 60 or more years. Obviously, each individual represents a variation on the regional and cultural constructions of masculinity that in turn represents variations on dominate and marginalized conceptions of masculinity within socioeconomic and regional cultures (Sabo, 2004; Connell, 1987). Marginalized constructs of masculinity are those manifested by some members of oppressed and least acceptable groups in our American society. Race, socioeconomic status, possible geographical location, and sexual preference all represent possible marginalized constructs of what constitutes "maleness." The federal and state laws establishing procedures and standards most often reflect the dominate white upper middle class, heterosexual constructs of "manhood." Recall that these men came into "manhood" in the 1940s through the early 1960s and express these earlier notions of what it means to be a "man."

In rural communities of Appalachia studied in this inquiry, nearly every man has some connection to coal mining. "Coal Miners," as they like to be called even after leaving the job, are stoic and proud of their profession. These men represent, for the most part, the dominant constructs of masculinity in Appalachia coal country. These men are known for their physical endurance and working with dangerous situations every day of their lives. Their attitude is that it is the man who goes into the mines and the women stay home to care for them and the children. These men see themselves as independent, tough and in no need of help of any kind. When they need assistance they want their wives to provide the care. In many cases the wife is physically unable to do these functions and it takes considerable skill to work out acceptable alternatives. The men of this region are reported by APS workers to be particularly stubborn about accepting any service that is voluntary. This is similar across urban and rural settings where many services must be accepted voluntarily by the men who are not obligated to accept the care or service.

In contrast, there is a diverse population within urban areas. There are men who have lived in the region all their lives as well as an increasing number of men who have moved from other areas to retire with their wives. They represent a wide range of working backgrounds and regional cultures. Yet, these men have the same overriding construction of what it means to be a man in this world, even though they have had many different ways of arriving at that internalized construct.

In both the rural Appalachian and urban settings considered in this inquiry, the notion of manliness and masculinity played an important role in the efforts of social service workers to locate and engage men in services. Most reports came from outsiders or members of the family. Very few reports were made by the men themselves. These reports were, for the most part, denied and refuted by many of the men. The notion that "real men" do not need help is one of the significant features of identifying and working with men in both settings.

DEFINITIONS OF MALE ELDER ABUSE IN APS AGENCIES

Elder abuse of men falls under APS mandates that include a wide range of disabilities and circumstances with individuals age 18 and above. Therefore APS workers have only a small number of elderly clients as compared to the total number of clients seen under the APS guidelines. Workers in both rural and urban settings similarly described general APS guidelines and descriptions of various forms of neglect, physical abuse, psychological/emotional abuse, financial/material abuse and medication abuse. For example, neglect is described in terms of failing to provide for the necessities of life such as food, shelter, and clothing. This can be self-neglect or neglect caused by a caregiver. Physical abuse is described as any form of assault, threats, physical injury, sexual assault, forced confinement, among others. Psychological/emotional takes many forms such as making threats, seeking to frighten and intimidation. Financial/material abuse is described as misappropriated or unauthorized use of credit cards, stealing possessions in the form of money or objects owned by the abused, and different forms of fraud to gain access to money or funds. Medication abuse is described as misuse of prescribed medications by over-medication or failure to provide needed medications. Not often mentioned, but used in the National Elder Abuse Incidence Report (National Center on Elder Abuse, 1998), is the act of abandonment as a form of abuse, most often perpetrated on elderly men. These are very general and limited definitions of elder abuse. There are no specific descriptions of abuse that are particular to men.

It is important to note that all of these definitions suggest that an individual who is "incapacitated" in some way is likely to be harmed and exploited. This assumes incapacity and dependency that are not compatible with the usual notions of masculinity and thus have significant consequences when working with most males.

ABUSED MEN IN AN URBAN SETTING

The APS staff interviewed for this paper reported that about 14% of all cases called into the department were substantiated for abuse (or found in need of services). Of this abused group, approximately 10% were elderly males. The department has been keeping specific statistics on elderly abuse since 2003 that show 297 out of 807 men who were 60 years or older (or 36.8%) have been victims of neglect or abuse. Of this total number for elderly men, 192 of the abuse for men (or 64.7%) were substantiated.

The majority of situations reported for investigation of elderly men involved self-neglect. The interviewed staff estimated that about 70% of reported cases are the result of self-neglect. The vast majority of these cases were reported by family members (not living with the man), friends, neighbors, and, occasionally, medical personnel at a doctor's office. The next most frequent abuse report involves abuse by a caregiver at a life care facility or nursing home, or within a home where the older man had befriended a caregiver who had exploited him.

In the urban setting for this study, married couples retire to its warmer climate and often are without family, friends or affiliations with churches or social groups. When one or both become debilitated, it is sometimes difficult for them to receive needed services because of financial eligibility restrictions in public and some nonprofit services. Services are costly. Their children live far away and those children who live locally have jobs and are unable to provide day care services because of cost.

Unlike tax breaks for child care, there are none for the care of the elderly. One important service that has helped, in some circumstances, is a for-profit group that is available at a minimum fee to manage financial problems and to help with paying bills. There are about 200 clients of APS who utilize this service in the urban setting.

In some cases, the man has become involved with a young woman who exploits through sexual favors or attention. One not so uncommon situation involves prostitutes exchanging services for access to the elderly man's credit card and cash. This type of situation has resulted in debts in the tens of thousands of dollars. In many of these cases the man does not want any interference from APS.

ABUSED OLDER MEN IN RURAL SETTINGS

An increasing number of elderly men in rural Appalachian communities are being exploited because of the drug addictions of family members, caretakers, young female addicts and prostitutes. The increasing population of the elderly in these communities makes them easy targets for exploitation. Many of the elderly men were involved in coal mining or related service jobs, and often these men were injured on the job. There has been a rise in cancer and work-related illnesses among these men who are often treated at home with strong pain killers.

Many of these elderly men have good retirement benefits from the United Mine Workers Association insurance which allow them to have access to doctors, hospitals and prescription medication. With the introduction of OxyContin, a narcotic oxycodone, known in the Appalachian region as "Hillbilly Heroin," as well as lesser narcotics, many men are being exploited, either by having their funds taken from them for these drugs or having the actual drugs themselves taken by caregivers and others. Due to the changes in their health and lifestyles, elderly men are increasingly treated for depression and anxiety. Fast acting drugs, such as Xanax, Valium and Ativan, intended to give relief in short time frames are also attractive to addicts who can exploit the elderly men.

At some point in their treatment and recovery, these men require assistance with daily tasks. Primarily in rural communities this need for assistance is filled by caregivers on a "word of mouth" basis, and most are not formally trained. Typically it has been found that these are women who have worked most of their lives cleaning homes, caring for elderly and other impaired individuals. Most are hard working, trustworthy women in their late 30s or 40s. These women usually have grown children who often assist them. Most of the arrangements are made through families or friends, and few if any organizations are involved. In many cases, the younger people involved in these situations become the exploiter, preying on the elderly through mutual need–hers for drugs and money and his for comfort, attention and sexual favors. As a result, one could view this as a "victimless crime." In the long term, all too often the elderly male is financially exploited, fails to receive appropriate medical treatment and is left destitute, lonely and depressed. Increasingly, the elderly man is drawn into the same patterns of drug addiction as the exploiter.

An illustrative case involves a retired coal miner who had become a superintendent of a large mine and had saved a great deal of money. After retirement, he needed home care as a result of surgery. He was able to find a caregiver through local friends to help him through his convalescence. A trustworthy woman in her 40s who was known in the community was hired. Early in his recovery, his caretaker was called away to care for her own family. Her daughter, a young woman in her 20s, took her place. The man and the young daughter developed a relationship over the next few months which included her "borrowing money" from him, borrowing drugs and eventually her sharing his bed. In a six month period, prior to an intervention by the man's son, $200,000 was spent supporting not only the caretaker's addiction, but also the addiction of the elderly man. Once discovered, the man refused to file charges and his recovery now included admissions to a detox center. This situation may seem extreme given the amount of money exploited by this woman. However, cases where men are exploited for their drugs or money occur every day. People of Appalachia are known for being self-reliant, and suspicious of government interventions. Likewise, they take seriously relationships in their community and talking with outsiders can have potentially serious consequences. The obvious consequences of both of these factors can be seen in the day-to-day dilemmas of the APS workers attempt to assist elderly men.

APS WITHTIN AN ELDER ABUSE CONTEXT

Penhale and Parker (1999) describe the issues of power differentials in work with anyone subject to public scrutiny and intervention, and note that work in APS makes clear the need to be aware of the power differentials. The worker has discretionary power to intercede under legislative authority. Likewise, the client can, if able and aware of rights, refuse services just as they can accept the services offered. As Penhale and Parker (1999) state, most often

> Older people receive care rather than treatment. They are perceived and treated as passive recipients of care rather than active participants, centrally involved in an enterprise premised on partnership. This can be potentially doubly stigmatizing because a positive outcome is generally denied by such approaches. The emphasis is on outcome and content rather than the process. (p. 5)

The potential for elderly men is that this power differential and marginalization of the elderly man's construct of self as independent and self-sufficient plays an important part in the engagement with the APS worker. In general, males in the United States and the elderly of this inquiry; males who grew up in a different period of history and social norms, including gender and family roles and relationships; constitute a particular context that must be appreciated and respected if any collaborative engagement is going to take place between the system representatives and the men themselves.

It is not only the male who has lived out the dominant themes of what it means to be a "man" in this particular world, it is the APS worker and the system that can be only an expression of the same fundamental construct. Thus, APS workers bring with them beliefs about what constitutes aging, gender, family, manhood, womanhood, abuse, neglect and all that these mean as one listens to a report and begins to make judgments and plans to investigate the allegations, which in turn have been constructed within the same cultural contexts. The idea of men as "victims" of abuse or neglect is *not part* of our general view of men in our society and thus challenges even the most experienced APS workers to make the necessary adjustments in recognizing the vulnerability of elderly men. Significantly, the subtleties of cultural values and beliefs are most often covert and difficult to detect for anyone. What might appear as concern and "typical" or "objective" practice by the APS worker might actually reflect the subtle values and assumptions held about men and vulnerability.

Pritchard (2001) suggests just such responses to the elderly male clients in England. In her study, men were often not treated the same as female clients and allegations of abuse were not looked upon as seriously as those directed toward women. One complaint that was found in this study was the issue of inclusion or collaboration between the worker and the client. In many instances the men did not feel included in choices and decisions being made about their situation. Importantly, it was found that many men wanted to talk about the situation with someone and felt unsupported in not having anyone listen to what they had gone through (Pritchard, 2001). As this study was conducted in England, there were different cultural traditions. It is also obvious that from Pritchard's description of the men and their circumstances that there were many similarities with American cultural constructions of what constitutes "manhood" for the community and for the men themselves.

A PROTOCOL FOR ENGAGING OLDER MEN

Most importantly is the participation and collaborative partnerships established between a worker and an elderly client, man or woman. In this case, with elderly men, Valokivi (2004) provides a succinct conclusion from her research in Finland:

> To ensure participation in services, there should exist as an alliance between the client and the worker. Alliance means a mutual commitment to supporting the client's coping and to responding to his/her needs. The client should be truly heard and included in negotiations and decision-making, according to the aged person's caregiver's desire to participate or withdraw. . . Alliances are based on mutual trust, which is an empowering element in client work. (p. 203)

Paralleling these findings, Prichard (2001, p. 102) noted four main points from her interviews with elderly men who were involved with social services:

1. to talk about abuse (past and recent), life experiences, dilemmas and fears for the future, the resolution of loyalties which have been abused.
2. to be given practical information and advice about sources of help.
3. to be offered options about possible actions and outcomes.
4. to go at the "victim's" pace, respecting the stresses involved in disclosing one's failure to cope effectively with those who have abused, and with one's fears of future suffering and disappointment.

Both the regional APS offices in Appalachia used in this inquiry and the Department of Social Services in the urban center have been working on the development of a strengths-based and solution-focused model of practice within their agencies. As a result, common themes emerged to describe their practice with elderly men as well as other client groups. The following process has emerged for being potentially helpful with elderly men, and addresses the results of the findings from both rural and urban settings described above.

Preparation

It is important for workers to spend some time considering their own constructs about abuse and neglect, working with elderly individuals, and working with elderly male clients. Doing this in a group as part of training and as part of efforts to improve services can be very helpful. Most often we take for granted that we are "professionals" and in some ways immune to values and judgments, and become habituated to practicing in the same way with all those with whom we come in contact. The notion of "I have seen this one before" is not too uncommon. Keeping an edge on a razor is not easy with continuous use, just as keeping from getting jaded or complacent in our day-to-day efforts can wear our alertness and practice down. Keeping up with potential services that would engage the client in ways other than providing minimal care needs to be a continuous effort on the part of management, supervisors and workers. Weekly or biweekly group supervision as well as bringing in outside consultants to jostle us out of our patterns can be helpful in keeping workers and staff open to each new referral. Even though most workers and staff feel overwhelmed and "do not have the time" to meet on a regular basis, this small amount of time can bring renewed sharpness and hope to the job and make the work go better and quicker. At the start of each new report or contact, workers might stop for a moment and clear the mind of the tasks that they might be facing. They should prepare themselves to meet the client where he is and give the client "time" to take in what is happening. One needs to be present with the client and attuned to what they need at the moment (Pritchard, 2001).

Joining

The client needs to be reassured that the worker is not there to harm him in any way and, importantly, there is the need to relieve his fears of not having any say or control in what might happen. The client needs to start to know who the worker is as a person, one who is concerned with his well-being. Male clients were once very self-reliant and for many there is suspiciousness about "government" interfering in their lives. This is particularly true in the Appalachian "coal miner's" mind. This is important in terms of the worker's intention. If the partnership is well established then changes are more likely to be mutual decisions and not as fearful at a later point. This is not giving false hope but realistic first intentions. Reassuring the client that the worker wants to work with him to help make decisions about the validity of the reported abuse and later how to address the issues listed in the abuse or neglect report gives him permission to work through loyalty issues or fears of recrimination or retribution by a caregiver.

- For example: "I understand that you do not like having me come to see you like this. I know you do not like a government agency like mine involved in your personal business."
- "I need your help in deciding if this report I have to check out is correct."
- "I know your wife has always been able to manage to do what is needed until now when her own health is keeping her from continuing to do this for you. I am sure you trust her more than anyone else and want her to continue to help. What do you think needs to happen to be able to take a care of both your needs now?"

Starting where the client is, which might very well be anger and resentment at being what they might see as an intrusion, needs to be acknowledged. It is necessary to remember that the worker's arrival might be the very first time the client has been asked to view his situation as an "issue or concern." This recognition will take time and pacing. Taking the next step depends on coming to some agreement on what is or is not an issue. Asking what ideas the client has and what the client thinks needs to happen, so that he is maintaining a safe and secure home for himself while not placing himself in further jeopardy, is a very important step in acknowledgement of his potential predicament as it builds rapport and security. It is also important in being able to address the anxiety and fears of taking steps too fast.

Gaining trust through respect and appreciating the perspective of the client helps build a collaborative partnership which engages the client in making decisions and a sense of empowerment in the midst of a "disempowering" experience. This does not mean that the worker agrees with the actions or ideas expressed but that the worker appreciates the individual's perception and ideas as his own and important to him. These are the key elements that make up the possible motivation and actions taken or not taken by the client. Engaging the client as a partner who is the expert on his needs (to what ever extent he has the mental capacity to state them and participate in the process) is a very important step. The real challenge for the worker is to see each client, in this case an elderly man, as truly unique and not a particular type of case like all others in a particular category, and to build on this unique-ness in terms of personal and social strengths and resiliency. All of this reflects the cultural background of the client in terms of how his own sense of "being a man" has been constructed. The bottom line is that if the man has the ability to understand and is not incapacitated, he might not acknowledge that there is a problem and can reject any assistance at this point.

- For example: "Even though you do not think it is her business, what do you think the person who asked us to see you was concerned about? What do you think?"
- "I know, as a coal miner, you have faced many dangers and have worked very hard, it has not been easy. Now you are in another dif-ficult place. What do you think would make things better?
- "I know you must enjoy the attention of Anna. Sex is an important part of your life."

Collaborative Goals and Solutions

At this phase, it must be recognized that not all elderly men come from the same socioeconomic backgrounds. Some men are primarily from the middle class, held steady jobs, and raised a family. Others have been poor throughout their entire lives or have failed to maintain steady employment or family life. For these men the idea of "hope" or planning past "today" can be a hard concept for them to consider. Considering possibilities and small steps to a better situation, rather than causes for incrimination, can help these men move toward hopefulness and possi-bilities (that are restorative). Focus on possible goals and small steps to-ward those goals or better future is in recognition that no matter what position a man is found, he has survived to this point through his own skills and strengths. It is not to deny pain, fear and anguish but to turn at-tention on the strengths and resiliency that has kept the man going no matter what the conditions. The shift is in moving from appreciating the difficulties and fears to how he has been able to cope with them, to keep going, even if painful, from day-to-day.

Complimenting the client's ability to endure and sustain himself under these circumstances is important. Acknowledging the strengths and endurance of the male client is important; he has strengths of endurance and has managed to make it this far. This acknowledgement can, even in serious cases, create a sense of hope for the man. Likewise, acknowledging and complimenting the caregiver who can no longer undertake what she wants (and feels is her duty) to do, is important in "letting go" while maintaining respect.

- "Things look pretty tough. How have you managed to keep going this way? What have you done to take care of yourself as much as you have?"
- "How have you kept this from being a problem for you?"

Scaling

This is a powerful tool that enables the client and the worker to find a common ground of understanding about the circumstances, arriving at a motivation for change and taking actions that give a better mutual understanding and appreciation of the situation facing the client (De Jong & Berg, 2002). Using a scale of "1" to "10," the worker a can designate the "1" on the scale to represent the worst that things have ever been during this period of time when needing care and "10" representing that the issues or concerns have all gone and there are no more "problems" in terms of neglect and abuse to manage. The client then provides his own personal estimation of where he is at the present, giving the worker an opportunity to clarify the meaning of the rating and to ask further questions that deal with coping and potentially identifying new ways of managing the situation. For example:

- "You said you would place yourself at a '2' on the scale. Since you have described to me how difficult things have been, I was wondering what you have done to keep yourself at a '2' and not at a '1' or below lately? What would need to be different for you to stay a solid '2' or what would have to happen to move to a solid '3' on your scale?"

As discussed, there is not only a statement of appreciation of how the client views the situation but scaling can suggest ideas of strengths and resilience even in the hardest times. Importantly, scaling opens the door to collaboration around what the client believes needs to be done either by himself, others or by potential services. The same scale can be used to ask the man how confident he is that he will be able to take action, and how likely (compliance) he is to make that effort. For example:

- "On a scale of '1' to '10,' how confident are you that you will be able to do this for the next few days ['1' equals, no way, impossible and '10' represents very easy, no problem]. This can be followed up with such questions as "What will you need to do to keep yourself at a firm '4' on your scale?"

Compliments, Task and Follow-Up

It is not often that we are complimented for our efforts. Being complimented is a powerful affirmation, if it is done out of respect and with all sincerity and genuineness. It is not about "cheerleading" but represents a sincere appreciation of what a person can do given the circumstances of his life. A simple compliment is to appreciate that this man has worked in, for example, the coal mines all his life and has been "self-sufficient." This will permit the worker to enter into his life and let him talk with the worker about needing help in any form that might be taken. For example:

- "I appreciate how mad you are about this report and I appreciate your talking to me about this situation."
- "You have worked hard all your life and it can't be easy now that this has happened."
- "I appreciate your willingness to talk with me even though you see no problems."

When the process is carried out respectfully from a strengths-based and solution-focused perspective, it is easier to address the findings from the research described previously, and to implement the client-centered directives (strengths-based and solution-focused practice that is collaborative) used in this inquiry by both the Appalachian and urban social service agencies (DeJong & Berg, 2002; Saleebey, 2006; Turnell & Edwards, 1999). It is important to note that these social service directives are primarily designed for work with children. This inquiry has extrapolated these basic principles for working with abused elderly men.

CONCLUSION

Elderly men represent a small proportion of clients who come to the attention of APS workers. Although a small proportion, these men are acknowledged by the practitioners in both rural and urban settings as deserving the same respect and services as are all other recipients. The supervisors and line workers who participated in conversations around this inquiry expressed, for the most part, a sense of respect and caring for these men. Both urban and rural APS workers expressed similar concerns about the need for respect to be given to the men they must evaluate and with whom they work over time. All workers believed that most of the men needed to be able to talk. One male worker commented that it is important to "just listen, let them talk." Occasionally, female workers will need to deal with the flirtatious elderly male who may or may not take them seriously at first.

It is "estimated that only one out of fourteen incidents of elder abuse, excluding incidents of self-neglect, come to the attention of authorities" (Pillemer & Finkelhor, 1988, p. 52). From their study, and many others, it is evident that there is a serious issue facing the growing elderly population. Even though men comprise a relatively small proportion of all older persons reported as abused, it is evident that they may be even more underrepresented as a result of self-neglect, underreporting, and shear pride that prevents them from seeking services or accepting services.

There is also the important issue of potential gender bias in the form of cultural socialization of workers and the social service bureaucracy that reflects the cultural values leading to the belief that men "don't cry." Such a belief by APS workers inadvertently can be expressed in the actions of the workers and in agency policy. The potential of enhanced services being offered to elderly men in the communities involved in this inquiry is being developed through the training in strengths and solution-focused practice. This is in addition to enhanced self-awareness of societal and regional attitudes toward men and those of the male clients. Hopefully, this will enable staff to better engage men and to develop more effective treatment. A significant issue is related to drug addiction, and the misuse of medications is a major issue in rural communities, with resulting neglect and abuse by caregivers (and growing addictions among elderly males). The isolation of rural communities and residents from services for older persons makes elder care and services difficult to monitor and assure safe practices. Mistrust of government also contributes to the avoidance of available services. These systemic issues, as well as the approach workers take with elderly males, need to be considered in efforts to address the abuse and neglect of elderly men.

Both the rural communities and the urban community expressed concern that resources focused upon older persons are not seen as urgent as those spent on children. The ageism factor will be an increasing factor as our society ages with the "baby boomers" reaching retirement. In rural areas, the populations are aging even faster as the young people are leaving for jobs in urban areas. For elderly men, the situation is aggravated by their own desire for independence that reflects the culture and the construct of "being a man." Obviously, more needs to be done to help both aging men and women to better prepare for themselves, if they have the means. Institutional changes need to be on the agenda if our society is to respond to the increasing needs of an elderly population. In a society focused on youthfulness, self-interest and independence, this will be a difficult task. From an applied perspectives, the workers' shift to a strengths- and solution-focused practice might assist in important, and increasing, efforts to engage abused and neglected men in the helping process.

REFERENCES

Aitken, L., & Griffin, G. (1996). *Gender issues in elder abuse*. Thousand Oaks, CA: Sage.

Connell, R. W. (1987). *Gender and power*. Stanford: Stanford University Press.

Cook, P. W. (1997). *Abused men: The hidden side of domestic violence*. Westport, CT: Praeger.

DeJong, P., & Berg, I.K. (2002). *Interviewing for solutions* (2nd ed.). Pacific Grove, CA: Brooks/Cole.

International Longevity Center. (2005). *Ageism in America: The report cards for presentation at the 2005 White House Conference on Ageing*. New York: International Longevity Center.

Kosberg, J.I. (1998). Abuse of elderly men. *Journal of Elder Abuse & Neglect. 9*(3), 69-88.

National Center on Elder Abuse. (1998). *National elder abuse incidence study*. Retrieved November 3, 2006, from http://www.aoa.gov/eldfam/Elder_Rights/ Elder_ Abusereport-full.pdf

National Victims Assistance Academy (1996) Elderly victims of crime. In *National Victim Assistance Academy 1996*. Retrieved November 3, 2006, from http://www. ojp.gov/ovc/assist/nvaa/ch18eld.htm

Penhale, B., & Parker, J. (1999). Elder abuse and older men: Towards an understanding. *Strasborg, 7-8*, 1-12.

Pillemer, K. & Finkelhor, D. (1988). The prevalence of elder abuse: A random sample survey. *The Gerontologist, 28*, p. 52.

Pritchard, J. (2001). *Male victims of elder abuse*. London: Jessica Kingsley Publishers.

Sabo, D. (2004). Masculinities and men's health: Moving toward post-superman era prevention. In M.S. Kimmel & M.A. Messner (Eds.), *Men's lives* (6th ed.). Boston: Pearson.

Saleebey, D. (2006). *The strengths perspective in social work practice*. Boston: Allyn & Bacon.

Shakespeare, W. (2003). King Lear. In T. Stern (Ed.), *King Lear* (Globe Education and A Theater Arts Book) (p. 50). New York: Routledge. (Original work published 1605).

Valokivi, H. (2004). Participation and citizenship of elderly persons: User experiences from Finland. In A. Metteri, T. Kroger, A. Pohjola, & R. Pirkko-Liisa (Eds.), *Social work visions from around the globe* (pp. 181-207). Binghamton, NY: Haworth Press.

doi:10.1300/J084v19n01_11

Index

AA. *See* Alcoholics Anonymous (AA)
Aarts, P.G.H., 166
Abandonment, defined, 78
Abner, E., 29,34
Abuse
  defined, 78
  described, 113
  discriminatory, in England,
    116-118,117t
  elder. *See also* Older men
    APS within context of, 181-183
    risk assessment in, 20-21
  institutional, in England,
    116-118,117t
  intimate partner, of older men,
    considerations for assessment
    of risk, 7-27. *See also*
    Intimate partner abuse, of
    older men
  nursing home/institutional, of older
    men, vulnerabilities for,
    138-142
  of older men. *See* Older men,
    abuse of
  public, of older men, vulnerabilities
    for, 142-144
  sexual. *See also* Sexual abuse
    of older men residing in nursing
    homes. *See also* Nursing
    homes, older men in, sexual
    abuse of
      profile of, 29-45
  substance
    in IPA of older men, 16
    in older men, treatment of,
    167-168
Achieving Best Evidence, 120
Acid(s), zolendronic, for osteoporosis
    in elderly men, 68

Action on Elder Abuse, 113
Adult Protection Committees, 113
Adult Protective Services (APS), 30,
    78,79,156,158
  within elder abuse context, 181-183
  lessons from, 159
  male elder abuse in, definitions of,
    178-179
  programs of, 20
  rural, in abuse of elderly male
    clients, 173
  urban, in abuse of elderly male
    clients, 173
Ageism in America, 174
Alcoholics Anonymous (AA), 163
Alendronate, for osteoporosis in
    elderly men, 67
Alienation, fractured relationships
    leading to abuse of older men
    related to, 88-89
Allegation(s), false, abuse of older men
    and, 101-102
Altfeld, S.J., 89,91
American College of Rheumatology, 68
American Healthcare Management,
    104
American Psychological Association,
    135
Anetzberger, G.J., 20,82
Appalachia, 181
Applegate, J.W., 162
APS. *See* Adult Protective Services
    (APS)
Aquilino, W.S., 84,89
Archer, J., 11

Bachman, R., 137,140

Bachman-Prehn study, 140
Balance exercises, for osteoporosis in
        elderly men, 66-67
Barrick, C., 167
Barusch, A.S., 161
"Battered Husband Syndrome," 2
Beard, H., 135
Beaulieu, M., 157
Beck Depression Inventory, 52
"Being a Man," 176-178
Bengtson, V., 84,90
Bereavement, in older men, treatment
        of, 166-167
Beyond Existing, 111,122-126,123t
Bias, gender, 10
Bisphosphonates, oral, for
        osteoporosis, in elderly men,
        67
Blundo, R., 173
BMD. See Bone mineral density
        (BMD)
Bobbitt, L., 177
Bone density test, 65
Bone loss, pathophysiology of, 63
Bone mineral density (BMD), 63
Bouter, L.M., 145
Bowie, S., 2
Boxer, A.M., 81,85
Boxton, W., 129
British Crime Survey, 112
Brody, E.M., 85,92
Brothers, B.J., 2
Bullington, J., 173
Burgess, A.W., 33
Buri, H., 155

Calcitonin, for osteoporosis in elderly
        men, 68
Calcium supplementation, for
        osteoporosis in elderly men,
        67
California Highway Patrol, 104
Callahan, J., 142,143
Caregiver(s)

family, abuse of older men by,
        104-105
institutional, abuse of older men by,
        103-104
non-relative, abuse of older men by,
        102-103
Cecil, K., 29,34
Children, adult,
        personalities/characteristics
        of, fractured relationships
        leading to abuse of older men
        related to, 82-83
Cicirelli, V.G., 77,85
Civokic, R., 31
Clawson, J., 88-89
CLSC René Cassin, Elder Abuse
        Center of, 56
"Coal Miners," 177
Cognitive impairments, in IPA of older
        men, 13-15
Cohler, B.J., 85
Comijs, H.C., 145
Conger, R.D., 91
Connors, G.J., 167
Cook, J.A., 85
Cook, P.W., 99,177
Cook-Daniels, L., 138
Cooney, T., 89
Coronary artery disease, management
        of, gender as factor in, 51-52
Crittenden, J.A., 153

Daly, J.M., 155
Danger Assessment, in IPA
        assessment, 18-19
Daughtry, D., 160-161
Davidson, K., 87
de Shazer, S., 165,166
Delusional jealousy, 15
Department of Health, 111-112,116
Dependency, relationship, in IPA of
        older men, 16-17
Depression, in older men, treatment of,
        166-167

Desmarais, S.L., 7
DEXA scan. *See* Dual-energy x-ray absorptiometry (DEXA) scan
Dietz, T.L., 12
Dills, E., 105
Dills, L., 105
Dills, R., 105
Discriminatory abuse, in England, 116-118,117t
Divorce, neglect of older men related to, 89-90
Doheny, M., 167
Douglas, K.S., 7
Draucker, C.B., 164
Dual-energy x-ray absorptiometry (DEXA) scan, in bone mineral density evaluation, 65

EASI. *See* Elder Abuse Suspicion Index (EASI)
Economic exploitation, of older men, 100-101
Edelman, H., 81-82
Edwards, G., 101
Edwards, P., 165
Edwards, T., 101
Eggebeen, D.J., 89
Elder abuse
    APS within context of, 181-183
    risk assessment in, 20-21
Elder Abuse Center, of CLSC René Cassin, 56
Elder Abuse Suspicion Index (EASI), 48,54-57
Elderly
    defined, 30
    sexual abuse of, 31
Elderly male clients, abuse of, 173-191
    implications for, 176-178
    introduction to, 174-176
    in rural settings, 180-181
    in urban setting, 179-180

Elderly Men: Special Problems and Professional Challenges, 2
Engels, G.I., 163
England, older male victims of abuse in, 109-127. *See also* Older men, abuse of, in England
Estok, P.J., 167
Ethical issues, in interventions for abused older men, 157-158
Etidronate, for osteoporosis in elderly men, 68
Exercise(s)
    balance, for osteoporosis in elderly men, 66-67
    weight-bearing, for osteoporosis in elderly men, 66-67

False allegations, abuse of older men and, 101-102
Family caregivers, abuse of older men by, 104-105
Family members, vulnerability to abuse of older men by, 134-138
Father-child relationship
    conflict in, fractured relationships leading to abuse of older men related to, 85-86
    contact and quality of, fractured relationships leading to abuse of older men related to, 83-85
Fear, in IPA of older men, 12
Fingerman, K.L., 83-84
Finkelhor, D., 10,11,14,32,80,86, 144-145
Friedrich, M., 102
Friedrich, R., 102
Fulmer, T., 82,86,156

Ganong, L., 88-89
Gender, as determinant in primary care, 50-54

coronary artery disease, 51-52
  patient gender differences, 50-52
  physician's gender, 52-54
Gender bias, 10
Gender specificity research, challenges
      facing, 57
Gendered policies and practices, as
      factors in abuse of older men,
      129-151. *See also* Older men,
      abuse of, risk factors for
General Accounting Office (GAO)
      report, 31
Gerschick, T.J., 141
Glasser, B.C., 76
Golay, H., 101
Goodrich, C.S., 21,79
Gough, P.C., 129
Gregorian, 33
Grossman, S.F., 11

Haas, M.L., 61
Hagestad, G.O., 80
Halifax International Airport, 102
Hamilton, R., 156-157,159
Haringsma, R., 163
Hart, S.D., 22
Hartz, A.J., 155
Hawes, C., 31,141
Health Select Committee, 114
Heitzman, R., 104
Help seeking, older men and, 159-162
Herzog, A.R., 89
"Hillbilly Heroin," 180
*Historical, Clinical, Risk
      Management–20*, 9
Hodge, P., 143
Holt, M.G., 32
"Husband Survives the Lumps and Bumps
      of a New Marriage," 177
Hwalek, M., 79

Ibandronate, for osteoporosis in elderly
      men, 68
Illinois Risk Assessment Protocol, 79
Impairment(s)
  cognitive, in IPA of older men,
      13-14

physical, in IPA of older men, 14
In One Ear Out the Other, 125
Institutional abuse, in England,
      116-118,117t
Institutional caregivers, abuse of older
      men by, 103-104
International Society for Clinical
      Densitometry (ISCD), 65-66
Intimate partner abuse (IPA)
  among older persons, 10-11
  defined, 9
  gender bias and, 10
  of older men
  considerations for assessment of
      risk, 7-27
  introduction to, 8-9
  risk assessment for, 17-21
      Danger Assessment in, 18-19
      ODARA in, 19-20
      SARA in, 19
  risk factors for
      assessment of, 21
      cognitive impairments, 13-15
      fear, 12
      implications of, 22-23
      living situation, 13
      mental illness, 15
      perpetrator, 14-17
      physical impairments, 14
      relationship dependency, 16-17
      research directions for, 22-23
      social isolation, 13
      substance abuse, 16
  risk assessment in, 18-20
      spousal assault instruments in, 18
IPA. *See* Intimate partner abuse (IPA)
ISCD. *See* International Society for
      Clinical Densitometry
      (ISCD)
Isolation, social, in IPA of older men, 13

Jasinski, J.L., 12
Jealousy, delusional, 15
Jogerst, G.J., 155
Jonker, C., 145
Joseph Rowntree Foundation, 110,111
Journal of Couples Therapy, 2

Journal of Sociology and Social Welfare, 3
Joyner, T., 103-104

Kahan, F.S., 133,136
Kaiser, C.B., 104
Kay, D., 153
Kaye, L.W., 2,81,153
Keeton, S., 83,85
Kernsmith, P., 16
Kidder, T., 141
King Lear, 133,174
Klibanski, A., 62
Koff, T., 2
Kosberg, J.I., 1,79,81,131,136,175
Kropp, P.R., 22

Lachs, M., 137,140
Langer, N., 93
Lawton, L., 84,90,91
Leclerc, N., 157
Lewellen, W., 105
Linzer, N., 158
Lithwick, M., 47
Living situation, in IPA of older men, 13
Local Authority and Social Services Act of 1970, 111
Lundy, M., 11

Male Victims of Elder Abuse: Their Experiences and Needs, 2
Mangum, W., 3
Matza, D., 82
McCarthy, E., 162
McDavid, K., 101
McKinlay, J., 143
McNeely, R.L., 99
Medicaid Fraud Reports, 31
Medicare, 9
Meehl, P., 17

"Meeting the Needs of Older Men: Challenges for Those in Helping Professions," 3
Meloy, M., 137,140
Members of Parliament, 114
Mendiondo, M.S., 29,34
Mental and Physical Comportment Scales of the Short Form Health Survey, 54-55
Mental Capacity Act 2005, 118
Mental illness, in IPA of older men, 15
Messman, T., 144
Miller, A.S., 141
Mistreatment, of older men, defined, 154-155
Mitteness, L.S., 77,82-85
Moore, A.J., 75
Moore, K., 61
Mouton, C.P., 32,81

Nahmiash, D., 79
Nakonezny, P.A., 84,90
National Clearinghouse on Abuse in Later Life (NCALL), 30
National Elder Abuse Incidence Study, 13,42,75-97,136,175. *See also* Older men, abuse of, fractured relationships and
  background of, 76-78
  described, 78-79
  funding of, 78-79
National Elder Abuse Incident Report, 179
National Film Board, of Canada, 102
National Institutes of Health, 62
National Ombudsman Reporting System (NORS), 31
National Osteoporosis Risk Assessment (NORA), 62
National Research Council, 154
National Violence Against Women Surgery, 12

NCALL. *See* National Clearinghouse
    on Abuse in Later Life
    (NCALL)
Neglect
  defined, 78
  of older men, vulnerabilities for,
    142-144
  potential
    of older men, contexts for, 86-90
    theoretical perspectives on,
    90-92
Newspaper accounts of male elder
    abuse, 99-108. *See also* Older
    men, abuse of, newspaper
    accounts of
Newspaper Archive.com, 100
Nichols, T.L., 7
Nightmare, 125
Nikzad, 33
1988 National Survey of Families and
    Households, 89
1996 National Victim Assistance
    Academy report, 174-175
*No Secrets: Guidance on Developing
    and Implementing
    Multi-Agency Policies and
    Procedures to Protect
    Vulnerable Adults from
    Abuse*, 111-113
NORA. *See* National Osteoporosis
    Risk Assessment (NORA)
NORS. *See* National Ombudsman
    Reporting System (NORS)
Norton, M.C., 166
Nursing home(s), older men in, sexual
    abuse of
  described, 31,32
  findings on, 32-34
  literature on, 34
  profile of, 29-45
    introduction to, 30
  study of, 34-41,36t-40t
    discussion of, 41-44
    methods of, 35
    results of, 35-41,36t-40t

Nursing home/institutional abuse, of
    older men, vulnerabilities for,
    138-142
Nussbaum, J.F., 84
Nydegger, C.N., 77,82-85

ODARA. *See* Ontario Domestic
    Assault Risk Assessment
    (ODARA)
Ogrodniczuk, J.S., 164
Old Friends, 141
Older men
  abuse of. *See also* Elderly male
    clients, abuse of
    in APS agencies, definitions of,
    178-179
  concepts related to, 154-156
    mistreatment, 154-155
    perpetrator relationship to
    victim, 155
    risk factors, 155-156
  controversy of, 156
  detection of
    perspectives from family
    practice, 47-60
    introduction to, 48-49
    physician's role in, 49
    tool in, 54-57
  in England
    Beyond Existing in, 122-126,
    123t
    case examples, 119-121
    identification of, 112-114
    identifying and working with,
    109-127
    introduction to, 110
    prevalence of, 114-116,
    114t-116t
    problems in identification of,
    118-119
    research projects on, 110-112
    types of abuse, 116-118,117t
    working with, 121-122

fractured relationships and, 75-97.
*See also National Elder
Abuse Incidence Study*
alienation-related, 88-89
causes of, 80-86
  conflict in father-child
      relationship, 85-86
  contact and quality of
      father-child
      relationship, 83-85
  personalities/characteristics
      of adult children,
      82-83
  personalities/characteristics
      of men, 80-82
described, 78-80
divorce-related, 89-90
future study of, suggestions for,
  94
introduction to, 76
remarriage-related, 87-88
stepchildren-related, 88-89
by institutional caregivers, 103-104
interventions for, 153-172
  current services, 156-159
  ethical considerations in,
      157-158
  future directions in, 169-170
  implications for practice, 169
  introduction to, 154
  recommendations for, 168-170
  settings for, 163-165
  staffing for, 169
  traditions in, 157
  training for, 169
  types of, 162-168
      outcomes of, 166-168
males suspected of, characteristics
  of, 55-56
newspaper accounts of, 99-108
  economic exploitation, 100-101
  false allegations, 101-102
  family caregivers, 104-105
  institutional caregivers, 103-104
  introduction to, 100

non-relative caregivers, 102-103
by non-relative caregivers, 102-103
prevalence of
  from EASI, 55
  perspectives from family
      practice, 47-60
  introduction to, 48-49
  from social worker assessments,
      56-57
risk factors for, 155-156
  gendered policies and practices
      increasing, 129-151
  introduction to, 130-131
  theoretical consideration in,
      131-133
  vulnerabilities to
      to nursing home/institutional
          abuse, 138-142
      public abuse and neglect,
          142-144
bereavement in, treatment of,
  166-167
defined, 30
depression in, treatment of, 166-167
economic exploitation of, 100-101
engaging of, protocol for, 183-188
  collaborative goals and solutions
      in, 186-187
  compliments in, 188
  described, 183-184
  follow-up in, 188
  joining in, 184-186
  preparation in, 184
  scaling in, 187-188
  task in, 188
help seeking by, 159-162
IPA of, considerations for
      assessment of risk, 7-27. *See
      also* Intimate partner abuse
      (IPA), of older men
neglect of
  contexts for, 86-90
  potential for, theoretical
      perspectives on, 90-92

in nursing homes, sexual abuse of.
     See also Nursing homes,
     older men in, sexual abuse of
profile of, 29-45
osteoporosis in, 61-73. *See also*
     Osteoporosis, in elderly men
PTSD in, treatment of, 166
socialization of, 159-160
substance abuse in, treatment of,
     167-168
vulnerabilities of, abuse related to,
     133-144
   described, 135-136
   family members–related,
     134-138
   trusted others–related, 134-138
Older Men's Lives, 2
Older persons
   defined, 9
   IPA among, 10-11
One Flew Over the Cuckoo's Nest, 105
Ontario Domestic Assault Risk
     Assessment (ODARA), 18
   in IPA of older men, 19-20
Op Den Velde, W., 166
Oral bisphosphonates, for osteoporosis
     in elderly men, 67
Osteoblast(s), 63
Osteoclast(s), 63
Osteoporosis
   described, 62
   in elderly men, 61-73
     diagnosis of, accuracy of, 65-66,
        66t
     introduction to, 62-63
     measurement tools, 64-65,65t
     risk factors for, 64
     treatment of, 66-69
        calcium supplementation in, 67
        exercises in, 66-67
        future research on, 69-70
        non-pharmacological
           interventions, 66-67
        off-label pharmaceuticals in,
           68-69

     pharmacologic, 67-68
OxyContin, 180

Pagelow, M.D., 86
Pamidronate, for osteoporosis in
     elderly men, 68
Paris, B.E.C., 133,136
Parker, J., 181-182
Paulk, D.L., 160-161
Payne, B.K., 31,135
Penhale, B., 181-182
Perpetrator(s), in IPA of older men,
     risk factors for, 14-17
Perpetrator relationship to victim, in
     abuse of older men, 155
Personalities/characteristics, fractured
     relationships leading to abuse
     of older men related to, 80-82
Physical impairments, in IPA of older
     men, 14
Pillemer, K., 10,11,13,14,32,80,83,
     85,86,140,144-145
Post traumatic stress disorder (PTSD),
     in older men, treatment of,
     166
Pot, A.M., 145
Primary care, gender as determinant in,
     50-54
Pritchard, J., 2,48,79,81,109,
     134-136,174,182-183
ProQuest Newspapers, 100
PTSD. *See* Post traumatic stress
     disorder (PTSD)
Public abuse, of older men,
     vulnerabilities for, 142-144
Puente, D., 102-103

Quinn, K., 79

Ramsey-Klawsnik, H., 29,33-35
Reel, T., 137

Reeves, K.A., 7
Relationship(s), fractured, abuse of
    older men related to, 75-97.
    See also Older men, abuse of,
    fractured relationships and
Relationship dependency, in IPA of
    older men, 16-17
Remarriage, neglect of older men
    related to, 87-88
Research, gender specificity,
    challenges facing, 57
Reynolds, S., 136
Rhodes, M., 104
Richman, A., 165
Risedronate, for osteoporosis in elderly
    men, 67
Risk of Abuse Tool, 20
Rivlin, G., Judge, 101
Roberto, K.A., 33,35
Robison, J., 83,85
Rodgers, J.L., 84

Sabo, D., 176
Sacks, G., 136
Sanford-Rocket, D., 158
SARA guide. *See* Spousal Assault Risk
    Assessment (SARA) guide
SASU. *See* Sex Abuse Survey (SASU)
Scally, L., 165
Scheyett, A.M., 162
Schut, 87
*Screening Tools and Referral Protocol
    for Stopping Abuse Against
    Older Ohioians: A Guide for
    Service Providers*, 20
Sedlack, C.A., 167
Self-neglect, defined, 78
"Self-neglecting," 142
Sex Abuse Survey (SASU), 35
Sexual abuse
    of older men residing in nursing
        homes. *See also* Nursing
        homes, older men in, sexual
        abuse of

profile of, 29-45
    of older persons, 31
Shakespeare, W., 175
Silverstein, M., 84,90
Simons, R.L., 91
Smit, J.H., 145
Social isolation, in IPA of older men,
    13
Social Security, 105
Social worker(s), assessments of, elder
    abuse prevalence data from,
    56-57
Social Worker Evaluation (SWE), 56
Socialization, of men, 159-160
Spinhoven, P., 163
SPJ. *See* Structured professional
    judgment (SPJ)
Spousal assault instruments, in IPA
    assessment, 18
Spousal Assault Risk Assessment
    (SARA) guide, 18,19
St. Charles Claywest, St. Louis, 104
State Council on Elder Abuse and
    Neglect, 136
State of Georgia, 136
Steinman, 85
Steinmetz, S.K., 2,79,112
Stepchildren, neglect of older men
    related to, 88-89
Stewart, G., 102
Stewart, M., 102
Stratego, A., 102
Stratton, D.C., 75
Straus, M.A., 112
Strauss, A.L., 76
Strobe, 87
Structured professional judgment
    (SPJ), 18
Substance abuse
    in IPA of older men, 16
    in older men, treatment of, 167-168
Suitor, J.J., 13,83-85
SWE. *See* Social Worker Evaluation
    (SWE)
Sykes, G., 82

Tai Chi, for osteoporosis in elderly
        men, 66-67
Tatara, T., 32
Teaster, P.B., 29,33-35
Teriparatide, for osteoporosis in
        elderly men, 68
Testosterone replacement therapy, for
        osteoporosis in elderly men,
        68
"The Abuse of Elderly Men," 2
*The Abuse of Men: Trauma Begets
        Trauma*, 2
The Adult Protection Analysis Project,
        113
"The Invisibility of Older Men in
        Gerontology," 3
*The Needs of Older Women: Services
        for Victims of Elder Abuse*,
        110
"The Victimization of Elderly Men," 2
Thomas, J.L., 92
Thomas, R., 100-101
Thompson, E.H., Jr., 2,129
Tomita, S.K., 82
Tooms, M., 29,34
Trusted persons, vulnerability to abuse
        of older men by, 134-138
Tsai, S.-J., 15
2005 White House Conference on
        Aging, 174

Uhlenberg, P., 89
UK National Prevalence Study of the
        Mistreatment and Abuse of
        Older People, 114
United Mine Workers Association, 180
US Pension Benefit Guaranty
        Corporation, 143

VA. *See* Veterans' Administration
        (VA)

Vados, P., 101
Valokivi, H., 183
Van den Hoonaard, D.K., 84
Van Der Leeden, R., 163
Veterans' Administration (VA), 105,
        166
    lessons from, 158-159

Wahle, C., 129
Weber, E., 144
Webster, P.S., 89
Weight-bearing exercises, for
        osteoporosis in elderly men,
        66-67
Weiss, D., 47
Westley, C., 154-155
Whitbeck, L.B., 91
White House Conference on Aging,
        143
WHO. *See* World Health Organization
        (WHO)
Wilber, K., 136
Willard, K., 104
Williams, J.M., 167
Wilson, K., 165
Wolfson, C., 47
Wood, J., 165
World Health Organization (WHO),
        65,66
World War II, 166
Wright, J.D., 144

Yaffe, M.J., 47

Zeller, R.A., 167
Zolendronic acid, for osteoporosis in
        elderly men, 68

T - #0243 - 101024 - C0 - 212/152/12 [14] - CB - 9780789035417 - Gloss Lamination